Ashish Trivedi
Sneha Deokar
Anushree Matre

Salivary Gland Disorders

AF755471

LAP LAMBERT Academic Publishing

Imprint

Cover image: www.ingimage.com

Publisher:
LAP LAMBERT Academic Publishing
is a trademark of
Dodo Books Indian Ocean Ltd. and OmniScriptum S.R.L publishing group

120 High Road, East Finchley, London, N2 9ED, United Kingdom
Str. Armeneasca 28/1, office 1, Chisinau MD-2012, Republic of Moldova, Europe
Managing Directors: Ieva Konstantinova, Victoria Ursu
info@omniscriptum.com

Printed at: see last page
ISBN: 978-620-8-44439-6

Ashish Trivedi
Sneha Deokar
Anushree Matre

Salivary Gland Disorders

Salivary gland disorders

Introduction

Salivary glands:

'The oral cavity is a moist environment; a film of fluid called saliva constantly coats its inner surfaces and occupies the space between the lining oral mucosa and the teeth. Salivary function provides host protection, assists in the initiation of food and fluid intake, and enables communication through speech. In humans there are three pairs of major salivary glands - the parotid, submandibular, and sublingual - located out side oral cavity, encapsulated, and with extended duct system to discharge their secretions. There are also a multitude of smaller minor salivary glands - the labial, lingual, palatal, glossopalatine, and retromolar - located just below and within the mucous membranes, unencapsulated, and with short duct systems. Secretion of each major salivary gland is not the same. The parotid gland secretes a "watery" serous saliva rich in amylase, the submandibular gland produces more mucinous saliva, and the sublingual gland produces viscous saliva. Because of these variations, saliva found in the mouth is referred to as mixed. The composition of mixed saliva is not the simple additive sum of all salivary secretions, as many proteins are rapidly removed as they adhere to hydroxyapatite of teeth and to the oral mucosal surfaces.

Without adequate salivary output, oral and pharyngeal health declines along with a person's quality of life. Salivary dysfunction, however, is not a normal consequence of growing older, and is due to systemic diseases, medications, and head and neck radiotherapy. While complains of xerostomia may be indicative of salivary gland disorder, salivary diseases can present without symptoms. Therefore, routine examination of salivary function must be part of any head, neck and oral examination.

Health care professionals can play a vital role in identifying patients at risk for developing salivary dysfunction and should provide appropriate preventive and interceptive techniques that will help preserve a person's health, function, and quality of life.

FUNCTIONS OF SALIVA

Mixed saliva has many functions, the most obvious being protection of the oral cavity.

Protection;

The protective function of saliva is expressed in many ways. Saliva is a lubricant. Its glycoprotein content, which makes it mucinous, protects the lining mucosa by forming a barrier against noxious stimuli, microbial toxins, and minor trauma. Its fluid consistency also provides a mechanical washing action, which flushes away nonadherent bacterial and acellular debris from the mouth. In particular, the clearance of sugars from the mouth by saliva's washing action limits their availability to acidogenic plaque microorganisms. The calcium-binding proteins in saliva help to form salivary pellicle, which behaves as a protective membrane.

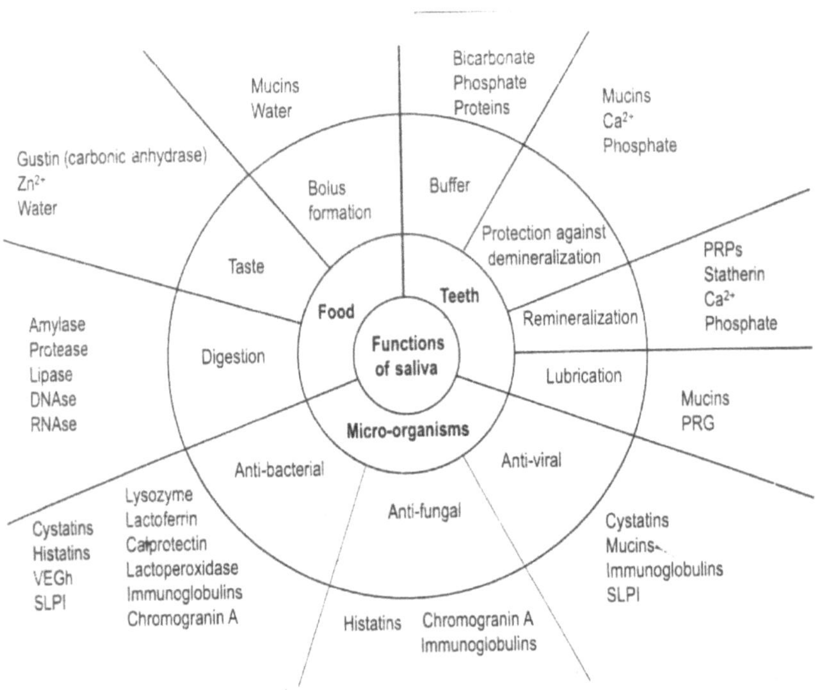

Buffering;

Saliva provides a buffer that protects the oral cavity in two ways: First, many bacteria require a specific pH for maximal growth; the buffering capacity of saliva prevents potential pathogens from colonizing the mouth by denying them optimal environmental conditions. Second, plaque microorganisms can produce acid from sugars, which, if not rapidly buffered and cleared by saliva, can demineralize enamel. Much of the buffering capacity of saliva resides in its bicarbonate and phosphate ions. Negatively charged residues on salivary proteins are also thought to serve as buffers; a salivary peptide, sialin, plays a significant role in raising the pH of dental plaque after exposure to fermentable carbohydrate. The ability of saliva to buffer acid is very important because saliva and plaque pH are generally lower in caries-active individuals.

Digestion;

Saliva is important for digestion. It provides taste acuity, neutralizes esophageal contents, dilutes gastric chime, forms the food bolous, and, because of its amylase contents, breaks down starch.

Taste;

Saliva also plays a role in taste. Although it enables the pleasurable sensations of food to be experienced, its primary role is protection in that it permits the recognition of noxious substances. Saliva is required to dissolve substances to be tasted and to carry them to the taste buds. It also contains a protein, called gustin, that is thought to be necessary for growth and maturation of the taste buds.

Antimicrobial Action;

Saliva has a major ecologic influence on the microorganisms that attempt to colonize oral tissues. In addition to the barrier effect of its mucus content, it contains a spectrum of proteins with antibacterial properties such as histatin. Lysozyme is an enzyme that can hydrolyze the cell walls of some bacteria. Lactoferrin binds free iron and in so doing deprives bacteria of this essential element. Antibodies are present in saliva. The major salivary immunoglobulin, secretory IgA, has the capacity to clump or agglutinate microorganisms. This ability, along with the cleansing action of saliva, serves to remove clumps of bacteria

Maintenance of Tooth Integrity;

Saliva is saturated with calcium and phosphate ions. The high concentration of these ions ensures that ionic exchange with the tooth surface is directed to the tooth. This exchange begins as soon as the tooth erupts because, although the crown is fully formed morphologically when it erupts, it is crystallographically incomplete. Interaction with saliva results in posteruptive maturation through diffusion of such ions as calcium, phosphorus, magnesium, and chloride into the surface apatite enamel crystals. Remineralization is achieved largely through the availability of phosphate and calcium ions in the saliva. If the fluoride ion is also available as remineralization occurs, the repaired lesion is less susceptible to future decay. On the other hand, saliva contains statherin, which inhibits calcium phosphate deposition as well as acidic proline-rich proteins which together with statherin, inhibits the growth of hydroscyapatite crystals.

Tissue Repair;

The clinical impression is that the bleeding time of oral tissue is shorter than that of other tissues. When saliva is experimentally mixed with blood, the clotting time may be greatly accelerated (although the resulting clot is less solid than normal). Experimental studies in mice have shown that the rate of wound contraction is significantly increased in the presence of saliva, which is thought due to the presence of epidermal growth factor in the saliva produced by the submandibular glands. The occurrence of growth factor is lower in human saliva, but its effect on repair has yet to be demonstrated.

Table 10.1: Functions of saliva, their mode of action and active agents

Functions	*Mode of action*	*Active agents*
1. Protection	• Lubrication • Lavage • Pellicle formation • Water proofing	• Glycoproteins • Water • Salivary protein and glycoprotein • Provide viscous somewhat waterproof layer on the surface of the teeth.
2. Digestion	• Bolus formation. • Digestion of starch. • Neutralization of esophageal contents	• Water • Amylase and alpha amylase enzymes • Phosphate and bicarbonate.
3. Buffering	• Maintenance of pH unsuitable for colonization of microorganisms. • Neutralization of acid.	• Phosphate and bicarbonate • Phosphate and bicarbonate
4. Taste	• Solution of molecules • Taste buds growth and maturation	• Water • Gusten
5. Antimicrobial	• Antibodies • Hostile environment • Barrier effect	• IgA, IgG and IgM • Lysozyme and lactoferrin • Glycoprotein
6. Tooth integrity	• Enamel maturation increases hardness, decreases permeability and increases resistance to caries. • Remineralization of the enamel lesions. • Decreased susceptibility: Repaired enamel lesions are less susceptible to future decay.	• Calcium and phosphate ions in saliva. • Calcium and phosphate ions in saliva. • When fluoride ions are also present in saliva, they get impregnated leading to acid resistant enamel.
7. Soft tissue repair	• Reduces bleeding time. • Rate of wound contraction is increased. • Rate of wound healing enhances. • Formation of blood clot.	• Active agent yet to be isolated probably viscosity of saliva also helps in checking bleeding • Epidermal growth factor produced by submandibular glands.

DEVELOPMENT OF THE SALIVARY GLANDS

The three major pairs of salivary glands - parotid, submandibular, and sub-lingual - originate uniformly from oral epithelial buds invading the underlying mesenchyme. The ectomesenchymal cells condense around this bud and to this point the sequence of events somewhat similar to initial tooth bud formation. The epithelial bud then clefts to form two or more new buds, and this process continues, producing successive generations and a hierarchical ramification of the gland. As in tooth development, ectomesenchyme plays a significant role in salivary gland development for both morphogenesis and cytodifferentiation of the gland. Various recombination experiments have shown that the presence of first arch ectomesenchyme is essential for full salivary gland development. For example, if nonsalivary gland mesenchyme is combined with salivary gland epithelium, the epithelium is maintained but does not differentiate into a glandular epithelium. However, when salivary gland ectomesenchyme is combined with pancreatic epithelium, pancreatic glandular cells differentiate. Such results indicate, again, the delicate interplay between epithelium and mesenchyme during development. All parenchymal (secretory) tissue of the glands arises from the proliferation of oral epithelium, which is either ectodermal (for the major glands) or endodermal (for the lingual glands) in origin. The stroma (capsule and septa) of the glands originates from mesenchyme that may be of either mesodermal or neural crest origin. In the case of salivary glands, the site of bud clefting is determined by the contraction of microfilaments within the epithelial cells, but the ordered deposition of collagen types I, III, and IV, laminin, and proteoglycan adjacent to the epithelial cells is also needed for further division of the bud to occur. In all the salivary glands, after the initial formation of the buds, the epithelial cell cord elongates to form the main duct primordium, which invades the sub epithelial stroma. At the distal end of this solid mass is a terminal bulb; this is the anlage of the intralobular salivary parenchyma. Branching produces arborization, and each branch terminates in one or two solid end bulbs. Elongation of the end bulbs follows, and lumina appear in their centers, transforming the end bulbs into terminal tubules. These tubules join the canalizing ducts (which are forming in the epithelial cord) to the peripheral acini. Canalization results from the mitosis of the outer layers of the cord being faster than that of the inner cell layers and canalization is completed prior to lumen formation beginning in the terminal bulbs. Necrosis or apoptosis of cord cells as a mechanism of canalization has never been observed. Canalization is complete by the 6th month post conception.

The development of a lumen within this branched epithelium generally occurs first in the distal end of the main cord and in branch cords, then in the proximal end of the main cord, and finally in the central portion of the main cord. Tubular lumenization is completed throughout the ductal tree before it occurs in the terminal buds. What determines the formation of the lumen is not known; however, it is not due, as has been suggested, to a separation of cells because of a buildup of secretory products from developing end pieces, because the cells have not yet formed, nor is programmed (apoptotic) cell death involved.

As lumina begin to appear in the terminal buds, the buds cleft and further subdivide into a series of unit's two cells thick called terminal saccules or terminal end pieces. It is within these terminal saccules that the secretory units develop, with the innermost cells differentiating into different types of secretory cells and some of the outer cells forming contractile myoepithelial cells. The epithelial component of the salivary gland (the parenchyma) is often likened to a bunch of grapes, with the ductal system representing the stalk stems and the terminal end pieces representing the grapes. Unlike a bunch of grapes, however, the salivary gland also has a connective tissue component that is rapidly diminishes as the parenchyma expands (terminal end pieces alone eventually occupy more than 90% of the gland); even so every terminal end piece and every duct remain supported by a tenuous connective tissue component carrying blood vessels and nerves. The final disposition of connective tissue is a capsule and septa that divide the gland into lobes and lobules. Because the capsule of a salivary gland is the last component of the gland to differentiate, it is not uncommon to find misplaced salivary tissue entrapped within facial bones if there is excessive epithelial proliferation. The lining epithelium of the ducts, tubules, and acini differentiates both morphologically and functionally. Contractile myoepithelial cells arise from neural crest ectomesenchyme to surround the acini. Myoepithelial cells differentiate at the time of onset of fetal secretory activity in the acini and achieve their full complement coincident with completion of the adult acinar- intercalated duct pattern at 24 weeks post conception in the submandibular gland and 35 weeks in the parotid gland. Interaction between epithelia, mesenchyme, nerve, and blood vessels is necessary for complete functional salivary gland morphogenesis. Autonomic innervation of the parenchymal cells is a key event in the salivary gland development. Sympathetic- nerve stimulation is necessary for acinar differentiation whereas parasympathetic nerve stimulation is important for overall gland growth. There is less understanding of what determines the differentiation of cell types that go to make up a terminal end piece. Little is known about the development of blood supply to the salivary glands.

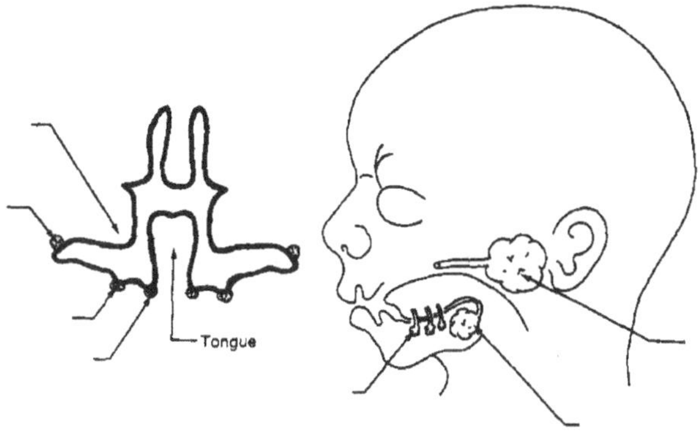

The parotid gland buds are the first to appear, at the 6th week after conception. They appear on the inner cheek near the angles of the mouth and then grow back to the ear. The maxillary and mandibular prominences merge, displacing the opening of the duct on the side of the cheek to some distance dorsally from the corner of the mouth. In the parotid or ear region, the epithelial cord of cells branches between the divisions of the facial nerve and to provide the acini and ducts of the gland. The ductal and acinar system is embedded in a mesenchymal stroma that is organized into lobules, and the whole gland becomes encapsulated by fibrous connective tissue. The parotid gland duct, repositioned upward, traces the path of the embryonic epithelial cord in the adult. The parotid ducts are canalized at 10 weeks post conception, the terminal buds are canalized at 16 weeks, and secretions commence at 18 weeks.

The submandibular salivary gland buds appear late in the 6th week as a grouped series, forming epithelial outgrowths on either side of the midline in the linguogingival groove of the floor of the mouth at the sites of the future papillae. An epithelial cord proliferates dorsally into the mesenchyme beneath the developing mylohyoid muscle, turning ventrally while branching and canalizing, to form the acini and duct of submandibular gland. Differentiation of the acini starts at 12 weeks; serous secretory activity starts at 16 weeks, increases until the 28th week, and then diminishes. The serous secretions during the 16th to 28th weeks contribute to the amniotic fluid and contain amylase and possibly nerve and epithelial growth factors. Growth of the submandibular gland continues postnatally with the formation of mucous acini. The mesenchymal stroma separates off the parenchymal lobules and provides the capsule of the gland.

The sublingual glands arise in the 8th week post conception as a series of about 10 epithelial buds just lateral to the submandibular gland anlagen. These branch and canalize to provide a number of ducts that open independently beneath the tongue. A great number of smaller salivary glands arise from the oral ectodermal and endodermal epithelium and remain as discrete acini and ducts scattered throughout the mouth. Labial salivary glands (on the inner aspect of the lip) arise during the 9th week post conception and are morphologically mature by the 25th week. Failure of bud canalization to form ducts before acinar salivary secretion commences results in retention cysts. Agenesis of the large salivary glands is rare.

STRUCTURE OF THE SALIVARY GLANDS

The description of salivary gland development makes it easy to appreciate that the parenchyma of the glands consists of a series of ducts ending in terminal secretory end pieces. The analogy to a bunch of grapes has already been presented, with the grapes representing the secretory end pieces and the stalks representing the duct system. Thus, following the pattern set by development, the main secretory duct of the salivary gland breaks up into a series of progressively smaller ducts (the striated ducts), which in turn branch into smaller intercalated ducts that open into the blind terminal secretory end pieces, which end as microvillus-lined canaliculi between the parenchymal cells. It is also easy to understand how every epithelial cell is supported by connective tissue, even though at times this is tenuous.

Terminal end pieces seen in section demonstrate great diversity in size, shape, and cell members. The shape of end pieces varies from simple circular outlines to tubular outlines to multilobed polygons. They consist of a collection of cells, polygonal in section, supported by a basement membrane that encloses a central space, the lumen. The intercellular spaces between the cells open into the lumina, and technically these spaces constitute the start of the ductal system. In serous glands (parotid) the cells in an end piece tend to be arranged in a roughly spherical form around a narrow lumen. In mucinous glands they tend to be arranged in a tubular or polygonal configuration with a larger central lumen.

Three cell types may be found in a terminal secretory end piece: mucous cells, serous cells, and myoepithelial cells. The number and distribution of each type of cell vary from gland to gland and from secretory end piece to secretory end piece.

The basement membrane is continuous around the terminal end piece and the ducts. It forms complex tubular scaffolding within which the epithelial cells are arranged, and it probably influences the maintenance of normal glandular architecture.

The terminal secretory end piece is also known as an acinus, but the use of this term is confusing. Past practice has been to refer to the spherical serous end piece as an acinus and to the mucus-secreting component end piece as a tubular secretory unit. When a tubular end piece is sectioned obliquely or transversely, however, the appearance of an acinus is created. If the term acinus is used to describe the morphology of the gland, it should be qualified as spherical acinus or tubular acinus.

The secretory cells in a salivary gland are classically described as either serous or mucous. Whereas they exhibit differing histologic features and their secretory products vary, the processes of synthesis and secretion arc similar.

Saliva is formed in the secretory end pieces and consists of two components: a macromolecular component derived from the synthetic and secretory activity of the acinar cells and a fluid component derived from the blood. Although the former process is reasonably well understood, the latter is less clear.

Formation of the Macromolecular Component;

The structure of the acinar cells is typical for cells involved in synthesis and secretion: abundant rough endoplasmic reticulum, prominent Golgi complexes, and numerous secretory vesicles. The Golgi complex plays a central role in synthesis and secretion - involved as it is in protein transport, concentration, and modification; secretory granule and lysosome formation; and the regulation of membrane traffic throughout the cell.

Proteins, synthesized in the rough endoplasmic reticulum, are shuttled to the Golgi complexes in transport vesicles, where after further modification they are packaged into secretory granules and then transferred to the cell surface where, after fusion of their unit membranes with the surface cell membranes and rupture, they are released to the external environment: a simple enough concept described as exocytosis, but one that involves a rather complicated process. As a secretory granule approaches the cell membrane, several events occur: removal of the web of microfilaments beneath the plasma membrane, fusion of the granule and cell membranes, rupture and rearrangement of the lipid layers of both to permit continuity of the granule membrane and cell membrane. Clearly this process, involving the addition of secretory granule membrane to plasma membrane, results in an overall increase in cell surface; thus a compensatory deletion mechanism must exist. Following the pharmacologically stimulated secretion of acinar cells, numerous small vesicles are found in the apical cytoplasm, indicating that endocytosis provides this compensatory mechanism. Indeed, when such vesicles are labeled they can be traced to lysosomes, the Golgi apparatus, or condensing vacuoles. This evidence, combined with biochemical evidence that the membrane surrounding the secretory granule derives from the Golgi apparatus and has a much longer half-life than the protein of the granule, provides clear proof for re - utilization.

Formation of the Fluid Component;

Salivary glands are able to secrete saliva equivalent to their own weight every 15 minutes for up to 1 hour when appropriately stimulated, and such a rate of secretion would not be possible if a filtration mechanism were responsible for fluid transport. After appropriate stimulation, it is thought that free Ca^{2+} is released from a storage site within the endoplasmic reticulum. Free cytoplasmic Ca^{2+} concentration can increase five- to tenfold in seconds after such stimulation, which brings about significant compensatory changes that include the opening of two membrane ion channels for passage of K^+ and C^{l-}, with the chlorine channel confined to the luminal surface of the cell and the potassium channel to the basolateral surface. When potassium is released from the cell, a compensatory uptake of Na^+ and Cl^- occurs. The Cl^- exits the cell through the channels at the luminal surface; it is speculated that, to maintain electrical neutrality, Na+ enters the lumen through the paracellular pathway. The result of these ionic relocations is a flux of water into the lumen via the osmotic coupling of NaCl and H20. Although the sodium chloride flux is reasonably well understood, the pathway for the flux of water has been debated, largely because, for a number of years, it was generally assumed that cell membranes exhibit low permeability to water. Recent studies on gallbladder epithelium, however, have shown that such cells are highly permeable to water and that the smallest changes in osmolarity are sufficient to drive large water fluxes. As a result, it is now thought that the production of salivary fluid also is a transcellular event.

Serous Cell;

The so-called serous cell in human salivary glands also secretes demonstrable amounts of polysaccharide, and therefore these cells are properly seromucous cells. Under the light microscope a seromucous cell is readily identifiable as pyramid shaped, with its apex situated towards the central lumen. Its nucleus is spherical and situated in the basal third of the cell. Its cytoplasm stains intensely with hematoxylin and eosin (H and E), giving the cell its characteristic basal hematoxyphilia. In well-fixed H and E-stained sections eosinophilic secretory granules about 1 micrometer in diameter are seen in the apical cytoplasm. With the increased resolution of an electron microscope, the seromucous cell has all the features of a cell specialized for the synthesis, storage, and secretion of protein. It has large amounts of rough endoplasmic reticulum arranged in parallel stacks packed basally and laterally to the nucleus. It also has a prominent Golgi complex situated either apically or laterally to the nucleus. Its apical cytoplasm is filled with secretory granules, each surrounded by a unit membrane. Similar to other cells, seromucous cells contain cytoplasmic organelles (e.g., mitochondria, found toward the lateral and basal portions of the cell, Lysosomes, free ribosomes, a few microbodies or Peroxisomes, microfilaments, and microtubules). It should be appreciated that his secretory process is continuous but cyclical, so that in any end piece seromucous cells at differing stages in the secretory cycle may be found. In a seromucous end piece, the cells are supported by a basement membrane that separates the parenchyma from connective tissue. The relationship between the basement membrane and the seromucous cell that it supports is complicated and varies. A straight relationship may exist, with both the basement membrane and the basal plasma membrane in close apposition, or the space between the basement membrane and basal plasma membrane may be increased by complex foldings of the basal plasma membrane, especially when the cell is not distended with secretory material. In the submandibular gland, seromucous cells possess a more complicated basal specialization than in the parotid gland. The plasma membrane is thrown into a series of tall, narrow basal folds extending beyond the lateral borders of the cell as foot processes that penetrate deeply into recesses in the folds of adjoining cells. Viewed from above, these cells have the appearance of multipointed stars. This specialization is estimated to increase the basal region of the cell by a factor of 60.

Laterally adjoining seromucous cells also have complex interrelationships. A well-defined intercellular space (or canaliculus) continues from the lumen of the end piece between these cells. The canaliculus terminates in the form of a classic junctional complex consisting of, in order, a tight junction (zonula occludens), an intermediate junction (zonula adherens), and a desmosome (macula adherens). At various points in this canalicular complex, apposing cells may contact and join in the form of desmosomal contacts and gap junctions. The surface of the seromucous cell, lining both the central lumen and the canaliculi, possesses delicate microvilli that extend into the luminal and canalicular spaces. The complex foldings of these cell surfaces are a reflection of their function of transporting fluid and electrolytes from the serum to saliva. Thus the seromucous cell is structurally adapted to fulfilling its varied purposes. Although the histology of all seromucous cells is fairly similar, it should be realized that physiologically the secretion of any seromucous cell may vary considerably. In fact, the granules of seromucous cells in the parotid, submandibular, and sublingual glands are morphologically all different, varying in electron density.

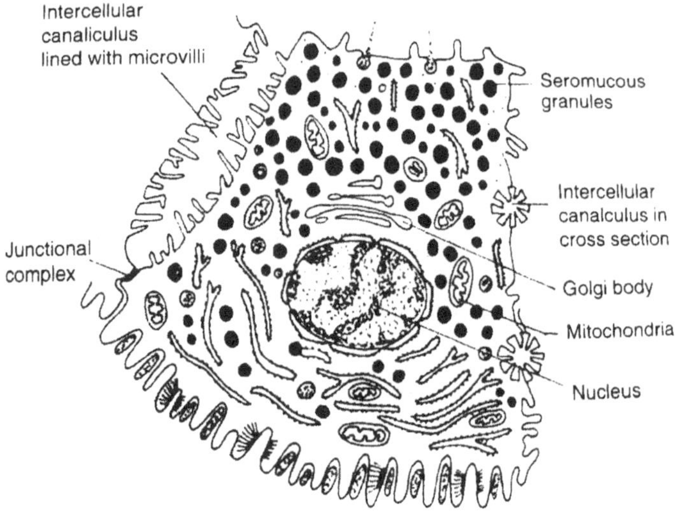

Mucous Cell;

The mucous cell is also well adapted for the production, storage, and secretion of proteinaceous material. Its secretory product differs from that of the seromucous cell in that there is a smaller enzymatic component and the proteins are linked to greater amounts of carbohydrate material-forming mucins. These differences are reflected in the structure of the cell. Under the light microscope, a mucous cell appears as pyramidal with a flattened nucleus situated toward its base. The apical portion of the cell does not stain strongly with H and E (in marked contrast to the seromucous cell) because of its higher carbohydrate content. Then again, if a mucous cell is stained specifically for carbohydrates, its apical cytoplasm stains intensely .Ultra structurally the mucous cell differs from the seromucous cell in that it contains more prominent Golgi complexes (which reflect the cell's increased carbohydrate metabolism) and its secretory material is stored in droplets. In resting cells, the rough endoplasmic reticulum and other cytoplasmic organelles (e.g., mitochondria) are less conspicuous than in seromucous cells and are mainly confined to the base and lateral aspects of the cell. The interdigitations between adjacent mucous cells tend to be fewer than between seromucous cells. Intercellular canaliculi are found leading to demilunes and also occur between mucous cells .In the submandibular and sublingual glands, mucous cells have a fairly complex system of basal folds, in the labial glands; mucous cells exhibit complex lateral interdigitations.

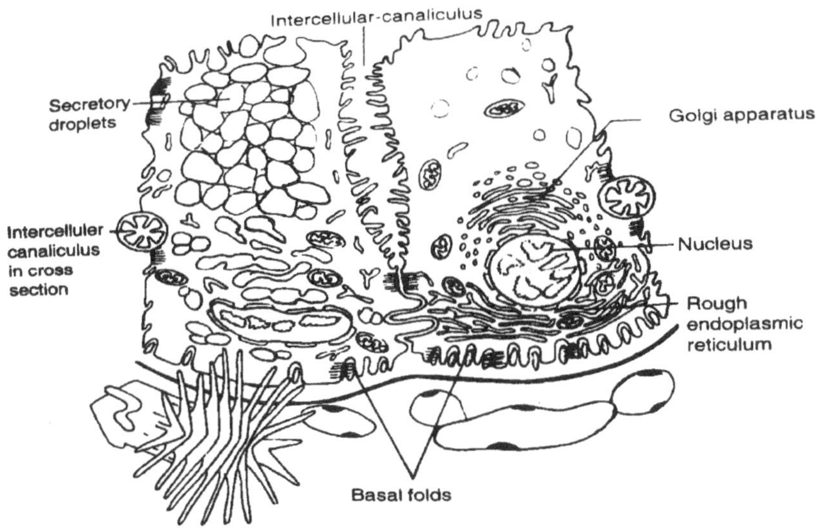

Secretory granules;

Both the seromucous and mucous cells package their products in secretory granules, and reference has been made to the structural variations of these granules. The variations are described as monopartite for granules containing a dense homogeneous matrix, bipartite for granules with a denser spherical inclusion, and tripartite for granules with a crescent-shaped component adhering to the inner surface of the membrane and enclosing the granule. Despite reports that such structural variations are confined to specific cell types in specific glands, all variations have been found in both seromucous and mucous cells of all glands. It has been suggested that these variations reflect the stage of maturation of the granule, but evidence is firmer that, because the secretory cells are able to produce a variety of proteins, these structural variations represent the proportional syntheses of different materials. The identification of a cell as seromucous or mucous by microscopy can be problematic because mucous cells at different stages of the functional cycle have different appearances. Thus a mucous cell at the beginning of its synthetic cycle may stain well with hematoxylin and eosin and closely resemble a seromucous cell. Recent studies taking this similarity into account have shown that the labial glands (previously regarded as mixed glands) are, in fact, mucous glands. Some of the mixed secretory end pieces in submandibular and sublingual glands could also be entirely mucous cells, but this has not been established.

Myoepithelial Cells;

The myoepithelial cell is found close to the terminal secretory end piece and the intercalated duct, occupying the space between basement membrane and basal plasma membrane of the secretory epithelial cells. There is usually one myoepithelial cell per secretory end piece, but two or three are not uncommon. Only their nuclei are visible in ordinary H and E-stained light microscope sections.

The morphology of a myoepithelial cell depends on its location. Cells associated with the secretory end pieces have been likened to an octopus sitting on a rock .Each cell consists of a central body (where the nucleus is situated) from which four to eight processes radiate and embrace the long axis of the secretory unit (from which other processes branch). The net effect is that the secretory end pieces are encompassed by processes of the myoepithelial cells running between the basement membrane and plasma membrane of the secretory cells in depressions on their surface. Desmosomal attachments are present between the myoepithelial cells and the underlying secretory cells to provide structural stability and prevent the processes from sliding over the acinar or duct cells during contraction. These processes contain many microfilaments (myofilaments) that frequently aggregate to form dark bodies along the course of the process. The microfilaments can be demonstrated by using immunofluorescence techniques to provide precise identification of myoepithelial cells in section. The normal cytoplasmic organdies found in any cell are mainly located in the perinuclear region of the cell. The cytoplasm has been described as sequestered into filamentous and nonfilamentous portions. The stromal surface of the cell has many invaginations containing neural fit that influence the cell's function. Myoepithelial cells related to the intercalated ducts in more spindle shaped and have fewer processes. On occasion, some are found with the cell body, situated in the intercalated duct region with processes extending backward as parts of the secretory end piece. The ultra structural features of myoepithelial cell are very similar to those of smooth muscle cells .The microfilaments, desmosomal attachments, and dark bodies are each found in myoepithelial cells as well as in smooth cells. Because of this similarity, myoepithelial cells are thought to have several possible functions, all related to the ability to contract. One function may be to act as a support for the secretory cells, preventing over distention as secretory products accumulate within the cytoplasm. Another may be to contract and widen the diameter of the intercalated ducts, thus lowering or raising their resistance to outflow. A third may be to aid in the rupture of acinar cells packed with mucus secretion. The origin of myoepithelial cells has not yet been determined. They are generally considered to be of epithelial origin because they are situated between the parenchymal cell and its basement membrane.

To recapitulate how the constituent cells are assembled to form end pieces of different morphology and function in any salivary gland, first is the spherical end piece consisting usually of seromucous cells. Second is the tubular end piece consisting of mucous cells intermixed with some seromucous cells and often capped by a crescent of seromucous cells, known as a demilune, that discharge their secretion into the tubular lumen via intercellular canaliculi running between the mucous cells. Third is the tubular end piece consisting solely of mucous cells. A salivary gland can therefore consist of a varied mixture of acinar and tubular secretory end pieces. Often whole lobules tend to consist of similar morphologic units.

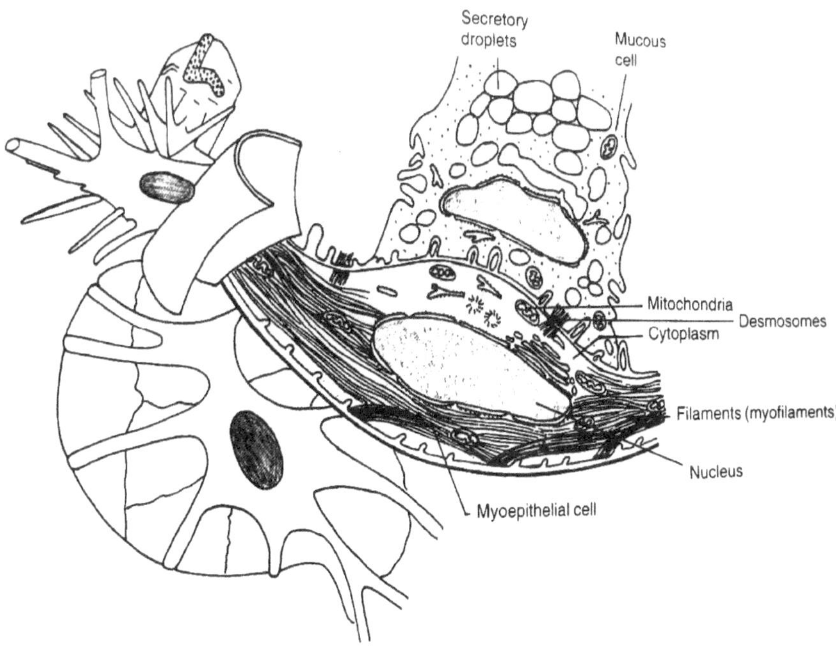

DUCTAL SYSTEM:

The ductal system of salivary glands is a varied network of ducts characterized by progressively smaller-diameter membranes. The network contains three classes of ducts: intercalated, striated, and terminal. The ductal system is not a simple conduit, for it actively participates in the production and modulation of saliva.

Intercalated Ducts;

The secretion of the terminal end pieces passes first through the intercalated ducts. These small-diameter ducts are lined by short, cuboidal cells with centrally placed nuclei and little cytoplasm, containing some rough endoplasmic reticulum situated basally and some Golgi complexes apically. Secretory granules are occasionally found in these cells, especially in cells closest to the secretory end pita. These cuboidal cells have a few microvilli projecting into the lumen of the duct, and their lateral borders interdigitate with each other and interconnect by means of junctional complexes situated apically, as well as by scattered desmosomal attachments below the junctional complexes, Myoepithelial cells, or their processes, are usually present between the basement membrane and the ductal cells. A high degree of structural pleomorphism has been described in the intercalated ducts of human labial and soft palate glands with respect to arrangement, location, length, diameter, and epithelial thick-ness within individual lobules. The simplest form of duct is lined by simple cuboidal epithelium. In human soft palate salivary glands, the intercalated ducts are usually relegated to connective tissue septa, are long and highly convoluted, ml consist of mucus-secreting cells, simple cuboidal epithelial cells, and myoepithelial cells. The functional activity of intercalated duct cells is not properly understood. Intercalated ducts are especially prominent in salivary glands with a serous secretion and therefore occur frequently in the parotid gland. They may be difficult to distinguish if embedded in a mass of secretory units.

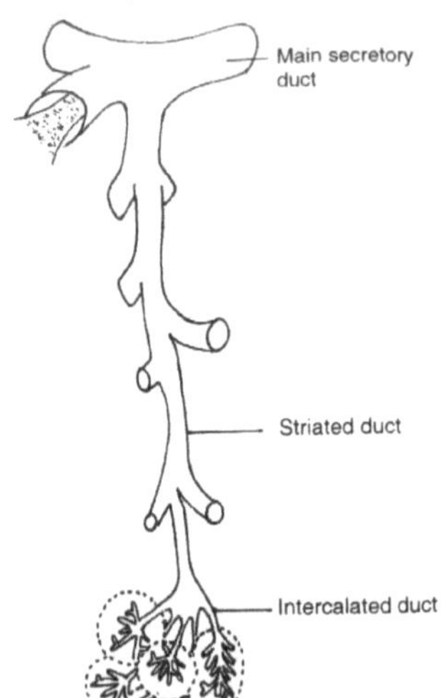

Striated Ducts;

The intercalated duct passes into the striated duct. Striated ducts are lined by columnar cells, which have centrally placed nuclei and intensely eosinophilic cytoplasm, making the duct clearly recognizable in H and E-stained sections. The most characteristic feature of such cells, however, is their prominent striations at the basal ends of the cells, giving the ducts their name. These striations are microscopy as particularly deep indentations of the basal plasma membrane into the cell .They also extend beyond the lateral boundaries of the cell as a series of foot processes that, in turn, possess complex secondary extensions. The lateral processes interlock in a highly complex fashion with adjacent cells and at the same time provides a large increase in the surface area of the basal plasma membrane. Many elongated mitochondria following the long axis of the folds occur in the cytoplasm between the folds. Around the nucleus are a few profiles of rough endoplasmic reticulum, along with some Golgi complexes. The apical cytoplasm often contains a few scattered vesicles, smooth endoplasmic reticulum, free ribosomes, and lysosomes. The luminal surface of the striated cell is characterized by short, stubby microvilli, and again adjacent cells are united by functional complexes and desmosomal attachments. Occasional dark cells containing numerous mitochondria and scattered small basal cells are usually also present. Striated ducts are always surrounded by a number of longitudinally oriented small blood vessels. Interspersed between the cells of the ductal epithelium of both intercalated and striated ducts are cells described simply as clear cell. They are thought to be of two types, one macrophage-like and the other lymphocytic, and both are involved in immune surveillance. The specialized structure of the striated ducts implies a particular function: They modify the secretions passing through them. Recall that this fluid is characterized by isotonic protein content, high sodium content (hypertonic), and low potassium content (hypotonic). As it passes along the striated duct, it changes to a generally hypotonic state. The massive infoldings of the basal plasma membrane, associated with the elongated mitochondria, are thought to reflect the sodium-pumping capacity of the cell wall in this location .Thus sodium, extracted from the cell, passes into the tissue fluid and establishes a concentration gradient between the cell and the luminar fluid. Sodium therefore diffuses into the cells from the luminal fluid; at the same time active transport of potassium occurs in the opposite direction. Bicarbonate ions are also actively secreted. Because under normal conditions of flow the striated duct cells do not absorb water, these ionic changes result in the formation of a hypotonic solution.

Excretory Ducts;

After passing through the striated ducts, salivary fluid is secreted into the oral cavity through the terminal excretory ducts. The histology of these ducts varies as they pass from the striated ducts to the oral cavity. Near the striated ducts they are lined by a pseudo stratified epithelium consisting of tall, columnar cells (much like striated cells) admixed with small basal cells; goblet cells also occur. As the terminal excretory ducts approach the oral cavity, their epithelium changes to a true stratified epithelium merging with that of the oral cavity at the ductal orifice. The main excretory ducts modify the final saliva by altering its electrolyte concentration, rendering it hypotonic, and perhaps also adding a mucoid component. Special eosinophilic cells, loaded with mitochondria, tend to be found in the ducts, particularly in mucosal glands. These cells, known as oncocytes, probably represent an age change. Regarding salivary gland parenchyma, one further observation needs to be made. Once development is completed, turnover of the parenchyma occurs, with continued replacement of acinar cells following their apoptotic deletion. This replacement is achieved by cell division at all sites within the parenchyma. That this is so has only recently been worked out; as a result, a number of theories to explain turnover exist, all linked to provide a satisfactory classification for salivary gland tumors.

CONNECTIVE TISSUE:

The connective tissue component of the salivary glands is the same as connective tissue elsewhere and comprises fibroblasts, macrophages, mast cells, adipose cells, and plasma cells, all embedded in an extra cellular matrix of collagen fibers and a ground substance of glycoproteins and proteoglycans. Oxytalan fibers are found in the submandibular and minor salivary glands. They are located in connective tissue supporting the mucous end pieces and around the smaller intralobular ducts and are thought to substitute for the elastic fibers that surround the larger extra lobular ducts. The connective tissue stroma of the salivary glands serves to carry the nerves and blood vessels (which are both highly specialized).

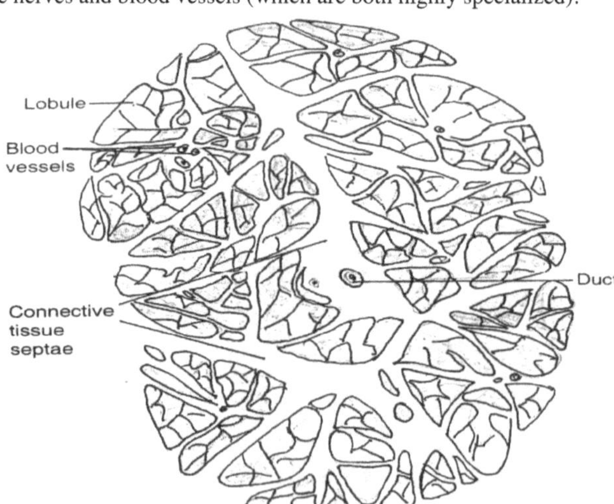

NERVE SUPPLY:

In most glands, secretory activity is controlled by impulses reaching the cells via secret motor nerves. In some glands, especially the smaller mucosal glands, a slow background of spontaneous secretion may occur independently of neural control. Salivary gland innervation is especially complicated; currently available information, obtained from the study of glands from many species, indicates that the glands receive postganglionic secret motor nerves from both sympathetic and parasympathetic sources, but there are wide variations among species, among the glands, and among cell types in the same gland. Despite these complexities in innervation patterns, it is possible to recognize (morphologically at least) two patterns of innervation. Nerves entering the salivary glands follow the blood vessels and break up into progressively smaller bundles until they form a final plexus adjacent to the terminal parenchyma. In this plexus the nerves consist of unmyelinated axons embedded in Schwann cell cytoplasm. From here, they are distributed to muscle arterioles, to secretory cells of the terminal end pieces, to myoepithelial cells, and to cells of the intercalated and striated ducts- It is now that the two patterns of innervation are established. In the first (described as epilemrrial), axons remain in the connective tissue separated from the secretory cells by the basement membrane. Where such axons come close to a secretory cell, they lose their Schwann cell covering, and in the adjacent exoplasm many vesicles containing transmitter substances exist. Presumably, some of the neurotransmitter substance is released when a nerve impulse passes and diffuses some 100 to 200 nm across the basement membrane before influencing the secretory cell. In the second (hypolemmal), axons penetrate the basement membrane, losing their Schwann cell covering in the process, and run between the secretory cells, separated from them by a gap of only 10 to 20 nni. Small headings occur along the course of these "bare" axons at sites where small vesicles and many mitochondria are often accumulated and where transmitter substance is considered to be principally released. With this type of innervation, a single axon may quickly affect several secretory cells or the small cell several times. In the ductal system, innervation is usually confined to the connective tissue. The flow of saliva is controlled entirely by nervous stimulation. Generally it is considered that /3-adrenergic (sympathetic) stimulation particularly induces protein secretory mechanisms, whereas L-adrenergic and cholinergic stimulation regulates water and electrolyte release. There is no direct inhibitory innervation of the salivary glands. The nervous "dry mouth," long thought to be the result of sympathetic inhibition as part of the fight or flight response, is explained by the direct inhibitory influence of higher centers on medullary centers.

In summary then, normal active reflex secretions of saliva involves the centrally coordinated formation of

1. Parasympathetic impulses, which tend to be more prevalent and

a. May occur in isolation

b. Usually evoke most of the fluid secreted

c. Cause variable degrees of exocytosis from some cells

d. Induce contraction of myoepithelial cells

e. Cause vasodilation as part of the secretory1 process

f. May have a direct influence on resynthesis

2. Sympathetic impulses, which are likely to occur more intermittently and

a. Act essentially on cells receiving parasympathetic impulses (and thus produce synergistic effects)

b. Often do not cause much mobilization of fluid

c. Tend to modulate the composition of saliva by increasing exocytosis from certain cells

Neurotransmitters;

Stimulation of cellular activity is achieved by the release of neurotransmitters, principally nor epinephrine and acetylcholine. These substances, found in small vesicular structures of approximately 40 nm diameter, appear agranular in cholinergic axons and granular in adrenergic axons. Scattered larger (80 to 1120 nm), dense-cored granular vesicles also occur in axons and are thought to be the site of various other neurotransmitter peptides such as substance P and Vasoactive intestinal peptide(VIP). Despite some evidence that the conventional transmitters are released in sub minimal amounts without any stimulation, when stimulated, neurons appear capable of releasing inexhaustible amounts of acetylcholine and nor epinephrine. However, the release of any neuropeptide requires high frequency stimulation, and its supply is soon exhausted. Regardless, when the neurotransmitter is released, it affects the parenchymal cell by binding with cell surface receptors and initiating further signaling mechanisms within the cell. Two such mechanisms occur: One involves the generation of cyclic adenosine monophosphate (AMP), and the other a breakdown of phosphatidylinositol-4, 5- biphosphate (with the breakdown products serving as intracellular messengers). Cyclic AMP generation results from adrenergic stimulation, which activates protein kinase to stimulate the secretion of protein, whereas cholinergic transmitters stimulate the second system, ultimately releasing free calcium (whose effect has already been described). It is also known that there is a salivary reflex involving periodontal receptors.

Finally, in addition to neurotransmitter regulation, hormones exert varying levels of salivary gland regulation. The hormones include estrogens, androgens, glucocorticoids, and peptide hormones. Although they can cause modification of salivary constituents, hormones cannot themselves initiate the flow of saliva. Myoepithelial cells contract because of impulses from both sympathetic and parasympathetic systems.

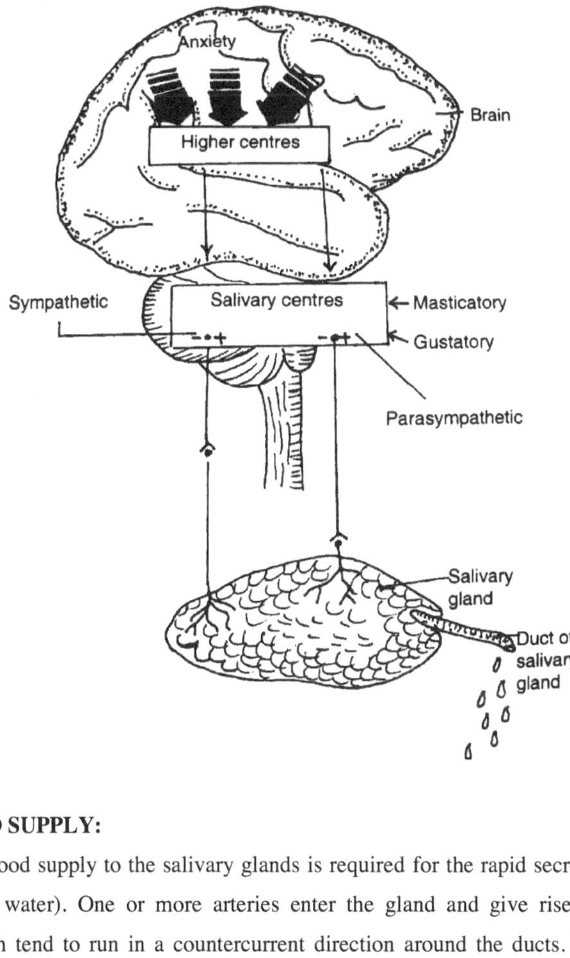

BLOOD SUPPLY:

An extensive blood supply to the salivary glands is required for the rapid secretion of saliva (which is 99% water). One or more arteries enter the gland and give rise to numerous arterioles, which tend to run in a countercurrent direction around the ducts. These vessels branch into a dense distribution of capillaries, particularly around the striated ducts. The distribution of capillaries around the secretory end pieces not as dense and takes the form of

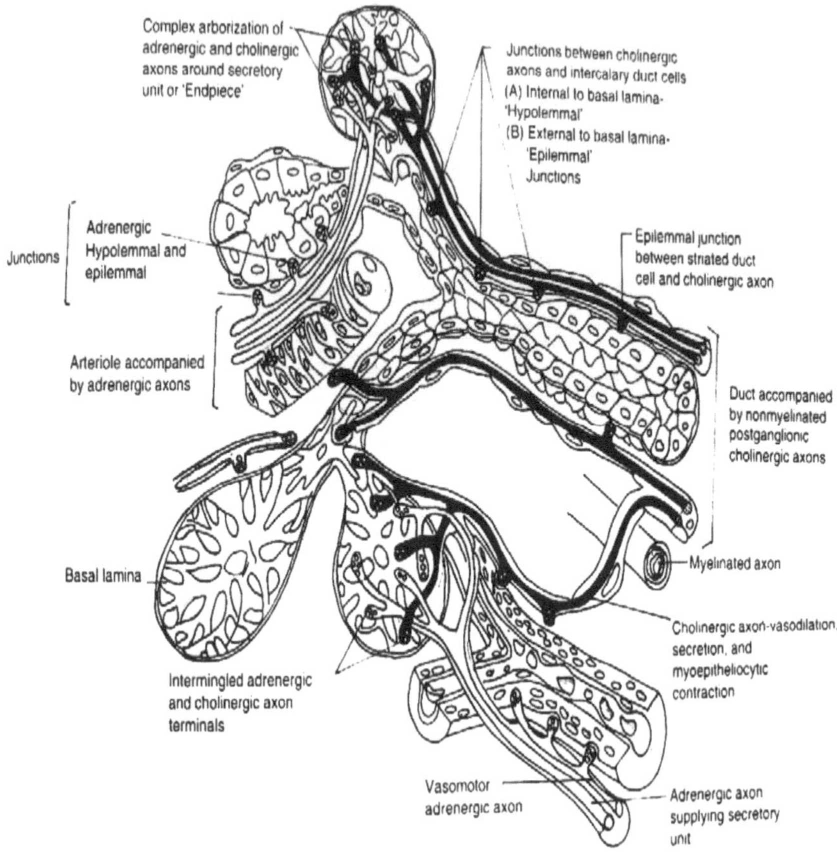

arterial arcades as the capillaries arise from the ends of the vessels supplying intralobular ducts. Venous return is accomplished by venea comnitantes as well as by larger veins that drain directly to the periphery of the gland. Arteriovenous anastomoses are found, related particularly to the acinar circulation. Definitive information concerning the lymphatic drainage is lacking. The pattern of microcirculation reflects the different functional components of a gland: A major concentration of capillaries is found around the striated ducts, where ionic exchange occurs; a lesser density occurs around the terminal secretory systems. A profound increase in blood flow normally accompanies salivary secretion.

ACE CHANGES:

Whether the salivary glands become less active with age is problematic, because such a great variation exists in the secretion of saliva. No longitudinal studies of salivary secretion on a single individual have thus far been reported. Even so, histologic changes associated with age have been reported within the salivary glands. Fatty degenerative changes, fibro-sis, and the progressive accumulation of lymphocytes in the salivary glands are thought to occur. Oncocytes—epithelial cells that can be identified by their marked granularity and acidophilia under the light microscope—are thought to represent an age change, although their significance has not been established. Ultra-structurally, they exhibit an accumulation of structurally altered mitochondria. Oncocytes are found in acini and in the intercalated and striated ducts of salivary glands, and they may give rise to neoplasms.

CLINICAL CONSIDERATIONS:

The rate of saliva production varies throughout the day. Of the 640 to 1200 ml secreted daily, only about 10 ml is produced at night. This nocturnal reduction in salivary secretion, along with the concomitant loss of its cleansing effect, is one reason why people should brush their teeth before retiring to bed. Developmental defects of salivary tissue are rare. Diagnostic techniques are now successfully applied to the readily available saliva, and saliva has also become a commonly used source of information regarding the metabolism and clearance of many drugs. In addition, biopsy of the labial gland is easily performed in the diagnosis of some systemic lesions. The most common conditions affecting the salivary glands are inflammatory disorders resulting from bacterial or viral infection (e.g., mumps). Painful swelling is then the usual symptom. Disease of the salivary glands usually brings about changes in the rate of salivary secretion and composition. These changes have a secondary effect in that they lead to the formation of plaque and calculus, which in turn has a direct bearing on the initiation of caries and periodontal disease. These diseases may become severe after therapeutic irradiation in and around the mouth. Because many systemic conditions (e.g., diabetes, cystic fibrosis) affect salivary flows, a patient complaining of dry mouth must be thoroughly investigated. . Obstructions to salivary flow may occur as a result of the formation of salivary calculi (stones) in the ducts, which tend to cause atrophy of the gland with an accompanying loss of function. The submandibular acinar cells often seem more re-sistant to such atrophic changes than the parotid glands, and the more mucinous glands (e.g., sublingual) are the most resistant. However, calculi occur most frequently in submandibular glands. Thus the type of gland determines the outcome of ductal obstruction.

MINOR SALIVARY GLANDS:

The minor salivary glands—lingual, buccal, and palatal—are small mucosal glands with short ducts that produce a primarily mucoprotein-rich secretion with a high secretory IgA concentration. The exception is the serous glands of von Ebner. The mucins from these glands come into close contact with the tooth and mucosal surfaces and as a result are important contributors to the protective mechanism of saliva. Because the minor salivary gland secretions are especially rich in mucosubstances, they are assumed to play an important role in the formation of acquired peliide. An interesting feature of the minor salivary glands is focal accumulation of lymphocytes around the duct walls; they are thought to have a role in the immune surveillance of the mouth.

SALIVARY GLAND ANATOMY AND PHYSIOLOGY

There are three major salivary glands: parotid, submandibular, and sublingual. These are paired glands that secrete highly modified saliva through a branching duct system. The parotid is the largest salivary gland. Situated in front of the ear and behind the ramus of the mandible, it weighs between 14 and 28 g and is intimately associated with peripheral branches of the facial nerve (VII). Parotid saliva is released through Stenson's duct, the orifice of which is visible on the buccal mucosa adjacent to the maxillary first molars. The duct runs forward across the masseter muscle and can easily be felt by moving a finger over the cheek when the jaws are clenched. At the anterior border of this muscle, the duct turns inward and opens into the oral cavity in a papilla opposite the maxillary first molar.

Next in size is the submandibular gland. Situated in the poster part of the floor of the mouth, tucked up against the medial aspect of the mandible, it weighs on average between l0 to 15g. It has an excretory duct that runs forward and opens into to the mouth beneath the tongue by way of a small orifice lateral to the lingual frenum.

The almond-shaped sublingual gland, the smallest of the three major salivary glands, weighs about 2 g and is situated in the floor of the mouth between the side of the tongue and the teeth.

Sublingual saliva may enter the floor of the mouth via a series of short independent ducts, but will empty into the submandibular (Wharton's) duct about half of the time. The orifice of Wharton's duct is located sublingually on either side of the lingual frenum. Often portions of the human sublingual and submandibular glands intermingle to form a gross sublingual-submandibular complex.

There are also thousands of minor salivary glands throughout the mouth, most of which are named for their anatomic location (labial, palatal, buccal, etc). These minor glands are located just below the mucosal surface and communicate with the oral cavity with short ducts. The minor salivary glands (estimated to be 600 to 1000) exist as small, discrete masses occupying the submucosa throughout most of the oral cavity. The only places where they do not occur are within the gingiva and in the anterior part of the hard palate. They are mucous glands, expect for the serous glands of von Ebner (which exist below the sulci of the circumvallate papillae and in the foliate papillae of tongue.

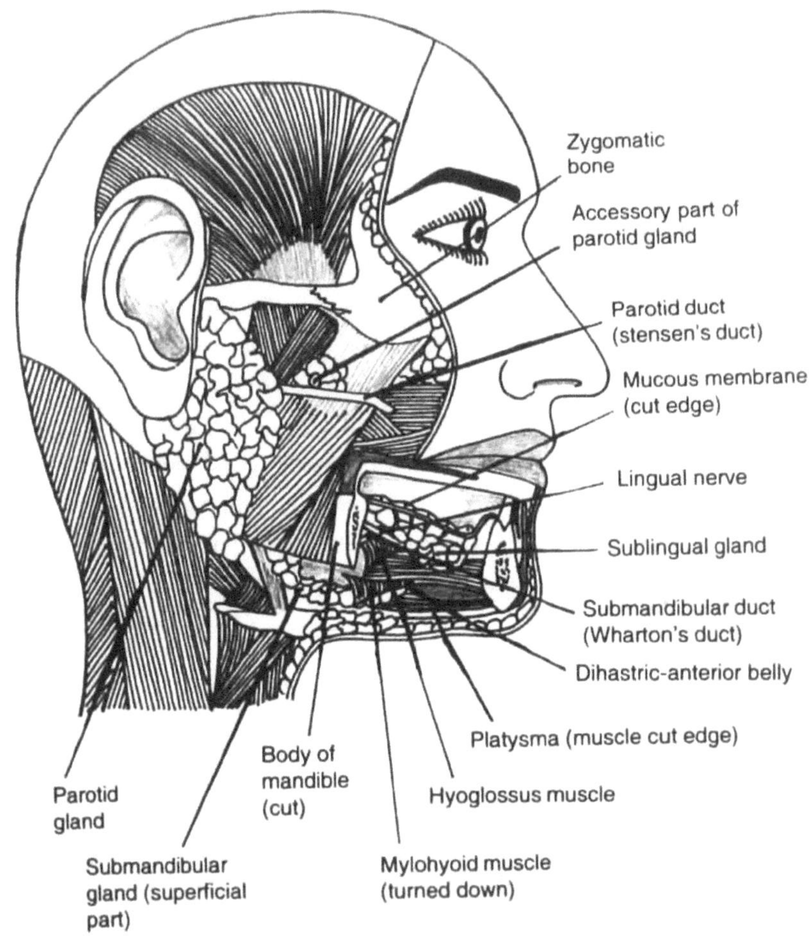

Saliva is the product of the major and minor salivary glands dispersed throughout the oral cavity. It is a highly complex mixture of water and organic and non-organic components. Most of the constituents are produced locally within the glands; others are transported from the circulation. The three major salivary glands share a basic anatomic structure. They are composed of acinar and ductal cells arranged much like a cluster of grapes on stems. The acinar cells (the "grapes" in this analogy) make up the secretory end piece and are the sole sites of fluid transport into the glands. The acinar cells of the parotid gland are serous, those of the sublingual gland are mucous, and those of the submandibular gland are of a mixed mucous and serous type. The duct cells (the "stems") form a branching system that carries the saliva from the acini into the oral cavity. The duct cell morphology changes as it progresses from the acinar junction toward the mouth, and different distinct regions can be identified. While fluid secretion occurs only through the acini, proteins are produced and transported into the saliva through both acinar and ductal cells. The primary saliva within the acinar end piece is isotonic with serum but undergoes extensive modification within the duct system, with resorption of sodium and chloride and secretion of potassium. The saliva, as it enters the oral cavity, is a protein-rich hypotonic fluid. The secretion of saliva is controlled by sympathetic and parasympathetic neural input. The stimulus for fluid secretion is primarily via muscarinic cholinergic receptors, and the stimulus for protein release occurs through β-adrenergic receptors. Ligation of these receptors induces a complex signaling and signal transduction pathway within the cells, involving numerous transport systems. An important point to consider is that loss of acini, as occurs in a number of clinical conditions, will limit the ability of the gland to transport fluid and to produce saliva. Also, muscarinic agonists will have the greatest effect in increasing saliva output as they are primarily responsible for the stimulus of fluid secretion. These points have implications for the treatment of salivary gland dysfunction.

DIAGNOSTIC APPROACHES TO THE PATIENT WITH SALIVARY GLAND DISEASE

Evaluation of Dry Mouth

The subjective feeling of oral dryness is termed xerostomia .Xerostomia is a symptom, not a diagnosis or disease. The term is used to encompass the spectrum of oral complaints voiced by patients with dry mouth. It is important to recognize that a patient complaining of dry mouth cannot automatically be assumed to have a salivary dysfunction. While oral dryness is most commonly the result of salivary gland dysfunction, it may have other causes. Patients need careful objective examination to identify the basis of their problem. Since individuals with salivary gland dysfunction are at risk for a variety of oral and systemic complications due to alterations in normal salivary performance, they should be identified, and appropriate treatment should be implemented. There are a number of non salivary causes of oral dryness complaints that should be considered, such as dehydration. Although dehydration may secondarily affect salivary gland output, changes in body water can affect mucosal hydration, which may lead to changes in the perception of wetness in the central cognitive alterations and oral sensory disturbances can lead to a sense of mucosal dryness. There are also psychological conditions that can lead to the complaint of dry mouth. Dysfunction of the salivary glands, however, is the most common cause of complaints of dry mouth. It is important to recognize that changes in salivary composition may be as important as a reduction in salivary output in some cases.

Therefore, the demonstration of seemingly adequate salivary flow alone is not a guarantee of normal salivary gland function .The differential diagnosis of xerostomia and salivary gland dysfunction is lengthy. The optimal approach to diagnosis is a sequential plan that first establishes the cause of the complaint, and then determines the extent of salivary gland hypo function that is present, and finally assesses the potential for treatment. An initial evaluation should include a past and present medical history, an oral examination, and an assessment of salivary function. Further techniques that may be indicated are salivary imaging, biopsy, and clinical laboratory assessment of hematologic variables. These are described below in more detail.

SYMPTOMS OF SALIVARY GLAND DYSFUNCTION

Symptoms in the patient with salivary gland hypofunction are related to decreased fluid in the oral cavity. Patients complain of dryness of all the oral mucosal surfaces, including the throat, and also of difficulty chewing, swallowing, and speaking. Many patients report a need to drink fluids while eating to help swallowing or report an inability to swallow dry foods. Most will carry fluids at all times for oral comfort and to aid speaking and swallowing. Pain is a common complaint. The mucosa may be sensitive to spicy or coarse foods, which limits the patient's enjoyment of meals.

PAST AND PRESENT MEDICAL HISTORY

A critical first step is a thorough history. If the past and present medical history reveals medical conditions or medications that are known to be associated with salivary gland dysfunction, a diagnosis may be obvious. Examples would be a patient who has received radiotherapy for a head and neck malignancy or an individual who has recently started taking a tri cyclic antidepressant. A recent survey found 1,500 drugs that are reported to have some incidence of dry mouth as a side effect. A complete history of all medications being taken (including over-the counter medications, supplements, and herbal preparations) is critical. Often the temporal association of symptom onset with the treatment is a valuable clue. When the history does not suggest an obvious diagnosis, further detailed exploration of the symptomatic complaint should be undertaken. Unfortunately, the general complaint of oral dryness is not well correlated with decreased salivary function, but specific symptoms may be.2 For example, while complaints of oral dryness at night or on awakening have not been found to be associated reliably with reduced salivary function, the complaints of oral dryness while eating, the need to sip liquids to swallow dry food, or difficulties in swallowing dry food have all been highly correlated with measured decreases in secretory capacity. These complaints focus on oral activities (eg, swallowing and eating) that rely on stimulated salivary function. Patients should also be questioned concerning dryness at other body sites. A patient's report of eye, throat, nasal, skin, or vaginal dryness, in addition to xerostomia, may be a significant indication of a systemic condition, such as Sjögren's syndrome.

CLINICAL EXAMINATION

Most patients with advanced salivary gland hypo function have obvious signs of mucosal dryness. The lips are often cracked, peeling, and atrophic. The buccal mucosa may be pale and corrugated in appearance, and the tongue may be smooth and reddened, with loss of papillation.

Patients may report that their lips stick to the teeth, and the oral mucosa may adhere to the dry enamel. There is often a marked increase in erosion and caries particularly decay on root surfaces and even cusp tip involvement. The decay may be progressive, even in the presence of vigilant oral hygiene. One should look for active caries and determine whether the caries' history and current condition are consistent with the patient's oral hygiene. While caries are unquestionably increased, it has not been determined definitively whether increased prevalence or severity of periodontal pathology is associated with salivary gland hypo function. Candidiasis, most commonly of the erythematous form, is frequent. Two additional indications of oral dryness that have been gleaned from clinical experience are the "lipstick" and "tongue blade" signs. In the former, the presence of lipstick or shed epithelial cells on the labial surfaces of the anterior maxillary teeth is indicative of reduced saliva (saliva would normally wet the mucosa and aid in cleansing the teeth). To test for the latter sign, the examiner can hold a tongue blade against the buccal mucosa; in a dry mouth, the tissue will adhere to the tongue blade as the blade is lifted away. Both signs suggest that the mucosa is not sufficiently moisturized by the saliva. Enlargement of the salivary glands is seen frequently. In these cases, one must distinguish between inflammatory, infectious, or neoplastic etiologies. The major salivary glands should be palpated to detect masses and also to determine if saliva can be expressed via the main excretory ducts. Normally, saliva can be expressed from each major gland orifice by compressing the glands with bimanual palpation and by pushing towards the orifice. The consistency of the secretions should be examined. The expressed saliva should be clear, watery, and copious. Viscous or scant secretions suggest chronically reduced function .A cloudy exudate may be a sign of bacterial infection although some patients with very low salivary function will have hazy flocculated secretions that are sterile. In these cases, there may be mucoid accretions and clumped epithelial cells, which lend the saliva a cloudy appearance. The exudate should be cultured if it does not appear clear, particularly in the case of an enlarged gland. Palpation should be painless. Enlarged painful glands are indicative of infection or acute inflammation. The consistency of the gland should be slightly rubbery but not hard, and distinct masses within the body of the gland should not be present.

SALIVA COLLECTION

Salivary flow rates provide essential information for diagnostic and research purposes. Salivary gland function should be determined by objective measurement techniques. Salivary flow rates can be calculated from the individual major salivary glands or from a mixed sample of the oral fluids, termed "whole saliva." Whole saliva is the mixed fluid contents of the mouth. The main methods of whole saliva collection include the draining, spitting, suction, and absorbent (swab) methods. The draining method is passive and requires the patient to allow saliva to flow from the mouth into a pre weighed test tube or graduated cylinder for a timed period. In the spitting method, the patient allows saliva to accumulate in the mouth and then expectorates into a pre weighed graduated cylinder, usually every 60 seconds for 2 to 5 minutes. The suction method uses an aspirator or saliva ejector to draw saliva from the mouth into a test tube for a defined time period. The absorbent method uses a pre weighed gauze sponge that is placed in the patient's mouth for a set amount of time. After collection, the sponge is weighed again, and the volume of saliva is determined gravimetrically. The suction and absorbent (swab) methods give a variable degree of stimulation of secretion and are therefore less reproducible. The draining and the spitting methods are more reliable and reproducible for unstimulated whole saliva collection. If a stimulated whole saliva collection is desired, a standardized method of stimulation should be used. Chewing unflavored gum base or an inert material such as paraffin wax or a rubber band at a controlled rate is a reliable and reproducible means of inducing saliva secretion. One can also apply 2% citric acid to the tongue at regular intervals. It is difficult to determine a "normal" value for salivary output as there is a large amount of interindividual variability and consequently a large range of normal values. However, with the collection methods described above, most experts do agree on the minimal values necessary to consider salivary output normal. Un stimulated whole saliva flow rates of < 0.1 mL/min and stimulated whole saliva flow rate's of < 1.0 mL/min are considered abnormally low and indicative of marked salivary hypo function. It is important to recognize that greater levels of output do not guarantee that function is normal. Indeed, they may represent marked hypo function for some individuals. These values represent a lower limit of normal and a guide for the clinician. Individual parotid gland saliva collection is performed by using Carlson-Crittenden collectors. The collectors are placed over the Stensen duct orifices and are held in place with gentle suction. Saliva from individual submandibular and sublingual glands is collected with an aspirating device or an alginate-held collector called a segregator. When using the suction device, gauze is placed sublingually to dry and isolate the sublingual region. The gauze and tongue are gently retracted away from the duct orifice. Gentle suction is used to collect the saliva as it is produced. The segregator is positioned over Wharton's ducts and is then held in place by alginate. As saliva is produced, it flows through tubing and is collected in a pre weighed vessel. Stimulated saliva from individual glands is obtained by applying a sialagogue such as citric acid to the dorsal surface of the tongue. Preweighed tubes are used for individual salivary gland collections and for some of the whole saliva collection techniques, and flow rates are determined gravimetrically in milliliters per minute per gland, assuming that the specific gravity of saliva is 1 (i.e., 1 g equals 1 mL of saliva). Samples to be retained for compositional analysis should be collected on ice and frozen until tested. Flow rates are affected by many factors. Patient position, hydration, diurnal variation, and time since stimulation can all affect salivary flow. Which ever technique is chosen for saliva collection, it is critical to use a well-defined, standardized, and clearly documented procedure. This allows meaningful comparisons to be made with other studies and with repeat measures in an individual over time. It is best to collect saliva in the morning. To insure an unstimulated sample, patients should refrain from eating, drinking, or smoking for 90 minutes prior to the collection. For a general assessment of salivary function, unstimulated whole saliva collection is the most valuable method of collection. It is easy to accomplish and is accurate and reproducible if carried out with a consistent and careful technique. Ideally, dentists would determine baseline values for unstimulated whole saliva output at an initial examination. This would allow later comparisons if patients begin to complain of oral dryness or present with other signs and symptoms of salivary dysfunction. For research purposes, or if more specific functional information is required for one particular gland, individual gland collection techniques should be used. These are not difficult but require specialized equipment and more time to accomplish.

SALIVARY GLAND IMAGING

A number of imaging techniques are useful in the evaluation of the salivary glands. For a full description of imaging techniques, depending on the technique used, imaging can provide information on salivary function, anatomic alterations, and space-occupying lesions within the glands. This section discusses plain film radiography, sialography, ultrasonography, radionuclide imaging, magnetic resonance imaging, and computed tomography

Plain-Film Radiography

Since the salivary glands are located relatively superficially, radiographic images may be obtained with standard dental radiographic techniques. Symptoms suggestive of salivary gland obstruction (swelling of the gland and pain) warrant plain-film radiography of the major salivary glands in order to visualize possible radiopaque sialoliths (stones) .Panoramic or lateral oblique and anteroposterior (AP) projections are used to visualize the parotid glands. Panoramic views overlap anatomic structures that can mask the presence of a salivary stone. A standard occlusal film can be placed intraorally adjacent to the parotid duct to visualize a stone close to the gland orifice. However, this technique will not capture the entire parotid gland. Sialoliths obstructing the submandibular gland can be visualized by panoramic, occlusal, or lateral oblique views. Smaller stones or poorly calcified sialoliths may not be visible radiographically. If a stone is not evident with plain-film radiography but clinical evaluation and history are suggestive of salivary gland obstruction, then additional images are necessary.

Sialography

Sialography is the radiographic visualization of the salivary gland following retrograde instillation of soluble contrast material into the ducts. Sialography is one of the oldest imaging procedures and was first mentioned by Carpy in 1902. In 1925, Barsony and Uslenghi separately described sialography as a diagnostic tool. Sialography is the recommended method for evaluating intrinsic and acquired abnormalities of the ductal system because it provides the clearest visualization of the branching ducts and acinar end pieces. Salivary ductal obstruction, whether by a sialolith or stricture, can be easily recognized by sialography. When patients present with a history of rapid-onset, acute, painful swelling of a single gland (typically brought on by eating), and sialography is the indicated imaging technique. Potential neoplasms are better visualized by cross-sectional imaging techniques such as computerized tomography or magnetic resonance imaging. The two contraindications to sialography are active infection and allergy to contrast media. Sialography performed during active infection may further irritate and potentially rupture the already inflamed gland. Additionally, the injection of contrast material might force bacteria throughout the ductal structure and worsen the infection. The iodine in the contrast media may induce an allergic reaction and also can interfere with thyroid function tests and with thyroid cancer.

Evaluation by nuclear medicine

Sialography can be performed on both the submandibular and parotid glands. Initial plain-film radiography is recommended for visualizing radiopaque stones and potential bony destruction from malignant lesions, as well as for providing a back ground for interpreting the sialogram. Oil- and water based contrast media are available. Both contain iodine and are therefore contraindicated in patients with iodine sensitivity. Oil-based contrast material is not diluted in saliva or absorbed across the mucosa, which allows for maximum opacificaton of the ductal and acinar structures. However, if extravasation into the glandular tissue occurs, the residual contrast material will remain at the site and may interfere with subsequent computed tomography (CT) images. Inflammatory responses and even the formation of granulomas have been reported following sialography using oil-based contrast. Injection of oil-based contrast medium requires more pressure because of its viscosity. Water-based dyes are soluble in saliva and can diffuse into the glandular tissue, which can result in decreased radiographic density and poor visualization of peripheral ducts, compared to oil-based contrast. Higher-viscosity water-soluble contrast agents that allow better visualization of the ductal structures are available and are recommended. Routine radiography includes panoramic, lateral oblique, AP, and "puffed-cheek" AP views. The normal ductal architecture has a "leafless tree" appearance. As the ductal structure branches through the major glands, the submandibular gland demonstrates a more abrupt transition in ductal diameter whereas the parotid gland demonstrates a gradual decrease in ductal diameter. Ductal stricture, obstruction, dilatation, ductal ruptures, and stones can be visualized by sialography. Non opaque sialoliths appear as voids. Sialectasis is the appearance of focal collections of contrast medium within the gland, seen in cases of sialadenitis and Sjögren's syndrome. The progression of severity is classified as punctate, globular, and cavitary. Sialography is the imaging technique of choice for delineating ductal anatomy and for identifying and localizing sialoliths. It also may be a valuable tool in presurgical planning prior to the removal of salivary masses. Following the procedure, the patient should be encouraged to massage the gland and/or to suck on lemon drops to promote the flow of saliva and contrast material out of the gland. Post procedure radiography is done approximately 1hour later. If a substantial amount of contrast material remains in the salivary gland at that time, follow-up visits should be scheduled until the contrast material empties or is fully resorbed. Incomplete clearing can be due to obstruction of salivary outflow, extraductal or extravasated contrast, collection of contrast material in abscess cavities, or impaired secretory function.

Ultrasonography

Due to their superficial locations, the parotid and submandibular glands are easily visualized by ultrasonography although the deep portion of the parotid gland is difficult to visualize because the mandibular ramus lies over the deep lobe. Ultrasonography is best at differentiating between intra- and extra glandular masses as well as between cystic and solid lesions. In general, solid benign lesions present as well-circumscribed hypo echoic intraglandular masses. Ultrasonography can demonstrate the presence of an abscess in an acutely inflamed gland, as well as the presence of sialoliths, which appear as echogenic densities that exhibit acoustic shadowing. Makula and colleagues studied a group of patients with Sjögren's syndrome and reported the appearance of parenchymal in homogeneity. They also noted good agreement between ultrasonographic, sialographic, and scintigraphic results in this patient group. Ultrasonography is a noninvasive and cost-effective imaging modality that can be used in the evaluation of masses occurring in the submandibular gland and the superficial lobe of the parotid gland.

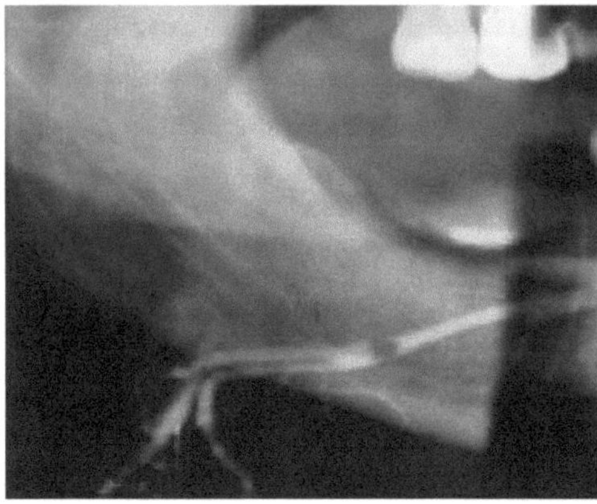

Radionuclide Salivary Imaging

Scintigraphy with technetium (Tc) 99m pertechnetate is a dynamic and minimally invasive diagnostic test to assess salivary gland function and to determine abnormalities in gland uptake and excretion. Scintigraphy is the only salivary imaging technique that provides information on the functional capabilities of the glands. Technetium is a pure gamma ray–emitting radionuclide that is taken up by the salivary glands (following intravenous injection), transported through the glands, and then secreted into the oral cavity. Uptake and secretion phases can be recognized on the scans. Uptake of Tc 99m by a salivary gland indicates that there is functional epithelial tissue present. The Tc-99m scan can be used as a measure of secretory function as it has been shown to correlate well with salivary output. Tc 99m is capable of substituting for chloride (Cl^-) in the sodium-potassium ($Na^+/K^+)/2Cl^-$ salivary transport pump and serves as a measurement of fluid movement in the salivary acinar glands. Duct cells can also accumulate Tc 99m. Scintigraphy is indicated for the evaluation of patients when sialography is contraindicated or cannot be performed (such as in cases of acute gland infection or iodine allergy) or when the major duct cannot be cannulated successfully. It has also been used to aid in the diagnosis of ductal obstruction, sialolithiasis, gland aplasia, Bell's palsy and Sjögren's syndrome. Salivary imaging is performed following the injection of 10 to 20 mCi of Tc 99m pertechnetate. The uptake, concentration, and excretion of the pertechnetate anion by the major salivary glands and other organs is imaged with a gamma detector that records both the number and the location of gamma particles released in a given field during a period of time. This information can be stored in a computer for later analysis or recorded directly on film from the gamma detector, to give static images.

Several rating scales exist for the evaluation of salivary scintiscans; however, no standard rating method presently exists. Current approaches to functional assessment include visual interpretation, time-activity curve analysis, and numeric indices. Most radiologists read Tc 99m scans by using visual interpretation and clinical judgment. A semi quantitative method exists in which Tc 99m uptake and secretion is calculated by computer analysis of a user-defined region of interest (ROI). Time-activity ROI studies are time-consuming and are more commonly used for research. Radionuclide imaging can provide information regarding salivary gland function by generating a time-activity curve.
A normal time-activity curve has three phases: flow, concentration, and washout. The flow phase is about 15 to 20 seconds in duration and represents the phase immediately following injection when the iostope is equilibrating in the blood and accumulating in the salivary gland at a sub maximal rate. The concentration phase represents the accumulation of Tc 99m pertechnetate in the gland through active transport. This phase starts about 1 minute after administration of the tracer and increases over the next 10 minutes. With normal salivary function, tracer activity should be apparent in the oral cavity without stimulation after 10 to 15 minutes. Approximately 15 minutes after administration, tracer begins to increase in the oral cavity and decrease in the salivary glands. A normal image should demonstrate uptake of Tc 99m by both the parotid and submandibular glands, and the uptake should be symmetrical. The last phase is the excretory or washout phase. During this phase, the patient is given a lemon drop, or citric acid is applied to the tongue to stimulate secretion. Normal clearing of Tc 99m should be prompt, uniform, and symmetrical. Activity remaining in the salivary glands after stimulation is suggestive of obstruction, certain tumors, and inflammation. With few exceptions, neoplasms arising within the salivary glands do not concentrate Tc 99m.However, Warthin's tumor and oncocytomas, which arise from ductal tissue, are capable of concentrating the tracer. They retain Tc 99m because they do not communicate with the ductal system, and they appear as areas of increased activity on static images. The difference is accentuated during the washout phase, when normal tissue activity decreases with stimulation and activity is retained in the tumors. Other salivary tumors may appear as areas of decreased activity on scintiscans.

Computed Tomography and Magnetic Resonance Imaging

Computed tomography (CT) images are produced by radiographic beams that penetrate the tissues .Computerized analysis of the variance of absorption produces a reconstructed image of the area. Coronal and axial images are usually obtained. The varying water content of tissues allows for magnetic resonance imaging (MRI) to distinguish tissue types .Tissues absorb and then re-emit electromagnetic energy when exposed to a strong electromagnetic field. Analysis of the net magnetization by radiofrequency is reconstructed to provide an image. Images are described as T1- or T2-weighted images, according to the rate constant with which magnetic polarization or relaxation occurs. CT and MRI are useful for evaluating salivary gland pathology, adjacent structures, and the proximity of salivary lesions to the facial nerve. The retromandibular vein, carotid artery, and deep lymph nodes also can be noted on CT. Osseous erosions and sclerosis are better visualized by CT than by MRI. Since calcified structures are better visualized by CT, this modality is especially useful for the evaluation of inflammatory conditions that are associated with sialoliths. Abscesses have a characteristic hyper vascular wall that is evident with CT imaging. CT also provides definition of cystic walls, making it possible to distinguish fluid-filled masses (i.e., cyst) from abscess.

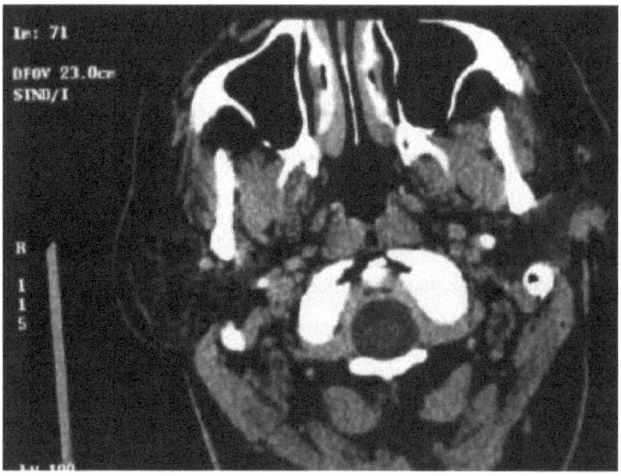

CT images of salivary glands should be obtained by using continuous fine cuts through the involved gland. Axial-plane cuts should include the superior aspect of the salivary glands, continuing to the hyoid bone and visualizing potentially enlarged lymph nodes in the suprahyoid neck region. Dental restorations may interfere with CT imaging and may require repositioning the patient to a semi axial position. Non-enhanced and enhanced CT images are routinely obtained. The initial non-enhanced scans are reviewed for the presence of sialoliths, masses, glandular enlargement and/or asymmetry, nodal involvement, and loss of tissue planes.

Glandular damage from chronic disease often alters the density of the salivary glands and makes the identification of masses more difficult. Contrast-enhanced images are more defined and accentuate pathology. Tumors, abscesses, and inflamed lymph nodes have abnormal enhancement compared to that of normal structures. Ultrafast CT and three-dimensional–image CT sialography have been reported by Szolar and colleagues to be an effective method of visualizing masses that are poorly defined on MRI; they also advocate Ultrafast CT for patients who are unable to lie still long enough for adequate MRI (pediatric, geriatric, claustrophobic, and mentally or physically challenged patients) and for patients for whom MRI is contraindicated. The disadvantages of CT include radiation exposure, administration of intravenous iodine-containing contrast media for enhancement, and potential scatter from dental restorations. MRI has become the imaging modality of choice for preoperative evaluation of salivary gland tumors because of its excellent ability to differentiate soft tissues and its ability to provide multiplanar imaging. It provides images for evaluating salivary gland pathology, adjacent structures, and proximity to the facial nerve. In T1-weighted images, the normal parotid gland has greater intensity than muscle and lower intensity than fat or subcutaneous tissue. In T2-weighted images, the parotid has greater intensity than adjacent muscle and lower intensity than fat. Structures and conditions that are dark on both T1- and T2-weighted images include calcifications, rapid blood flow, and fibrous tissue. The use of intravenous MRI contrast can improve imaging and aid in defining neoplastic processes, but its uses are specific, and indications should be discussed with the radiologist. MRI is preferred for salivary gland imaging because

(a) Patients are not exposed to radiation,

(b) No intravenous contrast media are required routinely, and

(c) There is minimal artifact from dental restorations.

MRI is contraindicated for patients with pacemakers or metallic implants such as aneurysmal bone clips. Patients who have difficulty maintaining a still position or patients with claustrophobia may have difficulty tolerating the MRI procedure, which may result in poor image quality.

SALIVARY GLAND BIOPSY

Definitive diagnosis of salivary pathology may require tissue examination. When Sjögren's syndrome is suspected, the labial minor salivary gland is the most frequently sampled site. This procedure is considered to be the most accurate sole criterion for diagnosis of the salivary component of this disorder. Standardized histopathologic grading systems are used to assess the extent of changes. Biopsy of minor glands can also be used to diagnose amyloidosis.

Biopsy of a minor gland of the lower lip is a minimal operative procedure that can be done with limited morbidity, using appropriate techniques. The incision is made on the inner aspect of the lower lip so that it is not externally visible. Six to ten minor gland lobules from just below the mucosal surface are removed and submitted for examination. The incision should be made through normal-appearing tissue, avoiding areas of trauma or inflammation of the lip that could influence the appearance of the underlying minor glands. Biopsy of the major salivary glands requires an extraoral approach. There is increased morbidity, and major gland biopsy has not been shown to offer diagnostic superiority to the minor gland procedure in patients with Sjögren's syndrome. When major gland biopsy is indicated, such as for the evaluation of a distinct salivary mass, fine-needle aspiration can be attempted. If this does not yield an adequate sample for diagnosis, an open biopsy procedure should be done. In cases of suspected lymphoma, immunophenotyping of the tissue is essential for diagnosis.

SEROLOGIC EVALUATION

Laboratory blood studies are helpful in the evaluation of dry mouth, particularly in suspected cases of Sjögren's syndrome. The presence of nonspecific markers of autoimmunity, such as antinuclear antibodies, rheumatoid factors, elevated immunoglobulins (particularly immunoglobulin G [IgG]), and erythrocyte sedimentation rate, or the presence of antibodies directed against the more specific extractable nuclear antigens SS-A/Ro or SS-B/La are important contributors to the definitive diagnosis of Sjögren's syndrome. Approximately 80% of patients with Sjögren's syndrome will display antinuclear antibodies, and about 60% will have antibodies against anti-SSA/ Ro. This latter autoantibody is considered the most specific marker for Sjögren's syndrome although it may be found in a small percentage of patients with systemic lupus erythematosus or other autoimmune connective-tissue disorders. Another serologic marker that may prove useful for the diagnosis of salivary gland disorders is serum amylase. This is frequently elevated in cases of salivary gland inflammation. Determination of amylase isoenzymes (pancreatic and salivary) will allow the recognition of salivary contributions to the total serum amylase concentration.

TABLE 9–1 Salivary Gland Imaging Modalities: Indications, Advantages, and Disadvantages

Imaging Modality	Indications	Advantages	Disadvantages
Ultrasonography	Biopsy guidance; mass detection	Noninvasive; cost-effective	No quantification of function; observer variability; limited visibility of deeper portions of gland; no morphologic information
Sialography	Stone, stricture; R/O autoimmune or radiation-induced sialadenitis	Visualizes ductal anatomy/ blockage	Invasive; requires iodine dye; no quantification
Radionuclide imaging	R/O autoimmune sialadenitis; sialosis, tumor	Quantification of function	Radiation exposure; no morphologic information
Computed tomography	R/O calcified structure; tumor	Differentiates osseous structures from soft tissue	No quantification; contrast dye injection; radiation exposure
Magnetic resonance imaging	R/O soft-tissue lesion	Soft-tissue resolution excellent, with ability to differentiate osseous structures from soft tissue; no radiation burden	Dental scatter; contraindicated with pacemaker or metal implant; no quantification

R/O = rule out

Evaluation of a Salivary Mass or Enlarged Salivary Gland

PRESENTATION

Salivary gland tumors most commonly present as an asymptomatic mass. Pain is not a reliable indicator of malignancy. Cystic enlargement, hemorrhage, or infection can cause pain in benign tumors. Malignant tumors often enlarge without symptoms, but when pain occurs, it is often the result of neural involvement and carries a worse prognosis. If nasal obstruction is also present, the clinician should suspect a tumor in the nasal or para nasal sinuses, possibly arising from a minor salivary gland.

PHYSICAL EXAMINATION OF THE SALIVARY GLANDS

The major salivary glands are palpated, and the orifices of the ducts are observed for saliva output. Normally, clear saliva should be expressed when the gland is pressed and "milked." The facial nerve is assessed for any decrease in motor function, and regional lymph nodes are palpated. Intraorally, any masses noted on the soft or hard palate are evaluated for ulceration of mucosa and invasion of associated structures. Tumors of the parotid gland will typically present as solitary painless mobile masses, most often located at the tail of the gland. It is important to document function of the facial nerve when evaluating parotid tumors, because the nerve runs through the gland, and evidence of decreased motor function of the nerve thus has diagnostic significance. Facial nerve paralysis is usually indicative of malignancy. Rarely, benign tumors may cause paralysis by either sudden rapid growth or the presence of an infection. Other findings suggesting malignancy include multiple masses, a fixed mass with invasion of surrounding tissue, and the presence of cervical lymphadenopathy. Tumors in the submandibular or sublingual glands usually present as painless solitary slow-growing mobile masses. Bimanual palpation, with one hand intraorally on the floor of the mouth and the other extraorally below the mandible, is necessary to evaluate the glands adequately. Tumors of the minor salivary glands are usually smooth masses located on the hard or soft palate. Ulceration of the overlying mucosa should raise suspicion of malignancy. Other lesions may mimic the presentation of salivary gland tumors.

Inflammatory diseases, infections, and nutritional deficiencies may present as diffuse glandular enlargement (usually of the parotid gland). Patients who are seropositive for human immunodeficiency virus (HIV) may develop cystic lymphoepithelial lesions that may be confused with tumors. Both melanoma and squamous cell carcinoma can metastasize to the parotid gland and appear similar to a primary salivary tumor. Chronic sialadenitis in the submandibular glands can commonly be confused with a tumor. In the minor salivary glands, necrotizing sialometaplasia can be confused with squamous cell carcinoma. This can have significant adverse consequences since the treatments for these two lesions are so different.

IMAGING

Plain-film radiography of the mandible or maxilla may be performed as a rapid and inexpensive way to determine if salivary tumors involve adjacent bony structures. The bone is assessed for compression by slow expansion or erosion by aggressive invasion. CT and MRI both image the salivary glands well, but they do not differentiate reliably between benign and malignant tumors. These modalities are not cost-effective for the initial evaluation of salivary gland lesions and are not recommended for the routine evaluation of salivary gland masses. Frequently, these imaging techniques are reserved for presurgical treatment planning, and initial evaluation is plain-film radiography followed by biopsy. If malignancy is known or suspected, scans can provide useful information about nodal involvement. Central necrosis of a lymph node is indicative of metastatic involvement. Technetium scanning is useful for diagnosing salivary gland tumors containing oncocytes, such as Warthin's tumor and oncocytoma. These lesions appear as bright masses on the scan, indicating active uptake and retention of the radionuclide. Technetium scanning also provides information on the functional capabilities of the major salivary glands.

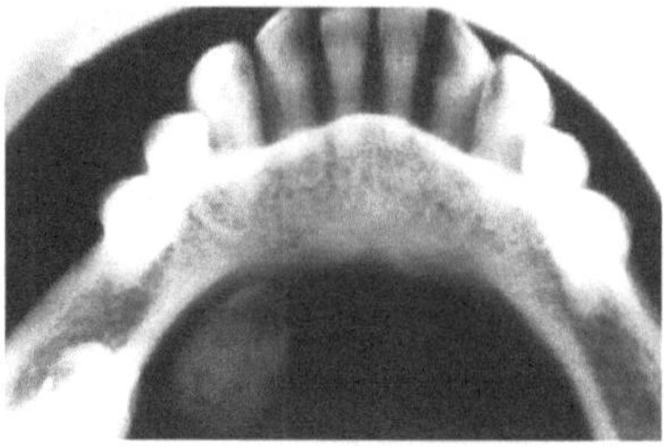

FINE-NEEDLE ASPIRATION BIOPSY

Fine-needle aspiration (FNA) biopsy is a simple and effective technique that aids the diagnosis of solid lesions. It may be particularly useful for elderly patients who can not tolerate an excisional biopsy because of medical considerations. A syringe is used to aspirate cells from the lesion for cytologic examination. To establish a diagnosis accurately, it is important to have a well-trained cytopathologist who is familiar with salivary cytology read the specimen. FNA biopsies do not provide a specimen with anatomic structure. The cytologist will examine the individual cells aspirated from the lesion and will offer a diagnosis based on the cellular characteristics of different lesions. Even if an exact diagnosis is not made, it may be possible to determine if a lesion is benign or malignant. Knowing the biologic aggressiveness of the tumor prior to definitive surgery is helpful in planning optimal treatment.

OPEN SURGICAL BIOPSY

A preoperative surgical biopsy is rarely indicated for salivary masses. In almost all salivary gland tumors, the treatment of choice is an excisional biopsy. In the parotid gland, this most often consists of a superficial parotidectomy, with careful preservation of the facial nerve. In small well-localized tumors of the parotid gland, local excision may be performed. Enucleation of tumors or local excision, however, is associated with a high recurrence rate in the parotid gland and is infrequently recommended. Tumors in the submandibular gland require the total removal of the gland. For tumors in the minor salivary glands, total excision with a margin of normal tissue is required. This approach is both diagnostic and curative in the majority of salivary gland tumors. Analysis of frozen sections should be performed at the time of surgery, to establish a diagnosis and guide the surgical approach. More than 80% of the time, the diagnosis based on the frozen section agrees with the final pathologic diagnosis from fixed and stained tissue. Most errors involve a failure to recognize malignant lesions. Malignant tumors are incorrectly called benign 5 to 24% of the time, but benign tumors are incorrectly diagnosed as malignant only 0 to 2% of the time. If frozen sections reveal a malignant tumor, the surgical margins may require extension.

STAGING OF SALIVARY GLAND TUMORS

A single tumor-node-metastasis (TNM) staging system is used for tumors of the parotid and submandibular glands. The letter "T" denotes tumor size as well as extension into adjacent tissue; the letter "N" indicates nodal involvement. Local lymph nodes that are commonly involved by tumors of the parotid gland include the intraparotid, intraauricular, and preauricular nodes. The submandibular gland drains locally to the submandibular, upper cervical and internal jugular lymph nodes. The letter "M" signifies metastases. Any nodal involvement other those mentioned above is considered a distant metastasis.

Staging for Major Salivary Gland Cancer

Tx Primary tumor cannot be assessed

To No evidence of primary tumor

T1 Tumor < 2 cm in greatest dimension

T2 Tumor 2–4 cm in greatest dimension

T3 Tumor 4–6 cm in greatest dimension

T4 Tumor >6 cm in greatest dimension

All categories are subdivided:

(a) No local extension,

(b) Local extension.

Local extension is clinical/macroscopic invasion of skin, soft tissue, bone or nerve.

Microscopic evidence alone is not considered local extension for classification purposes.

Nx Regional nodes cannot be assessed

N0 No regional lymph node metastases

N1 Single ipsilateral node < 3 cm in diameter

N2a Single ipsilateral node 3–6 cm in diameter

N2b Multiple ipsilateral node, none > 6 cm

N2C Bilateral or contra lateral nodes, none > 6 cm

N3 Metastasis in a lymph node > 6 cm

Mx Presence of distant metastases cannot be assessed

M0 No distant metastases

M1 Distant metastases

Stage I T1a N0 M0

T2a N0 M0

Stage II T1b N0 M0

T2b N0 M0

T3a N0 M0

Stage III T3b N0 M0

T4a N0 M0

Any T (except T4b) Nl M0

Stage IV T4b Any N M0

Any T N2N3 M0

Any T Any N M1

Adapted from the American Joint Committee for Cancer Staging and End Results Reporting: manual staging of cancer. Chicago 1988

Classification of salivary gland diseases

I. Developmental

1. Aplasia—absence of the gland
2. Atresia—absence of the duct
3. Aberrancy—ectopic gland

II. Enlargement of the gland

A. **Inflammatory**

1. Viral: Mumps, coxsackie A, CMV, echovirus, parainfluenza virus 1 and influenza virus
2. Bacterial
3. Allergic
4. Sarcoidosis
5. Obstructive

B. **Non-Inflammatory**

1. Autoimmune: Sjogren's syndrome and Mickulicz's disease
2. Alcoholic cirrhosis

3. Diabetes mellitus
4. Nutritional deficiency
5. HIV associated

III. Cysts

1. Extravasation cysts
2. Retention cysts
3. Ranula

IV. Tumours of salivary glands

A. **Benign tumours:**

1. Pleomorphic adenoma
2. Warthin's tumour
3. Basal cell adenoma
4. Myoepithelioma
5. Canalicular adenoma
6. Ductal papilloma

B. **Malignant tumours.**

i. Mucoepidermoid carcinoma
ii. Adenoid cystic carcinoma
iii. Malignant pleomorphic adenoma

V.Necrotizing sialometaplasia

VI. Salivary gland disfunction

1.Xerostomia
2.Sialorrhea

General and etiological classification of salivary gland disorders

A. General classification

1. Developmental anomalies:

a. Aplasia/agenesis
b. Atresia of ducts
c. Hypoplasia
d. Congenital fistula
e. Aberrancy
f. Accessory ducts and lobes.

2. Inflammatory (sialadenitis):

a. Bacterial: (i) acute (ii) chronic, (iii) recurrent parotitis of childhood

b. Specific infections.

c. Allergic.

d. Viral: (i) mumps (ii) salivary inclusion disease.

e. Post-irradiation

f. Sialadenitis of minor glands.

3. Obstructive and traumatic:

i. Papillary obstruction of duct

ii. Obstruction of duct lumen, e.g. sialolithiasis

iii. Obstruction due to changes in and around duct wall, e.g. strictures

iv. Salivary duct fistula

v. Frey's syndrome

vi. Mucocele (i) mucous extravasation cyst (ii) mucous retention cyst, (iii) ranula: (a) Superficial, (b) deep, (c) plunging

4. Changes in salivary secretion and composition in disease:

a. Functional disorders of salivary glands,

b. Factors influencing salivary flow rate,

c. Xerostomia/dry mouth.

5. Ptyalism (sialorrhea):

i. Acute inflammatory conditions, e.g. abscess, herpes infection, aphthae

ii. Tooth eruption

iii. Mental retardation

iv. Parkinsonism

v. Schizophrenia

vi. Epilepsy

vii. Mecury poisoning

viii. Acrodynia

ix. Rabies

x. Familial dysantonomia

6. Tumours and tumour-tike lesions: The revised WHO histological classification of salivary gland tumors and tumor-like lesions:

A. Adenoma:

(i) pleomorphic adenoma, (ii) Myoepithelioma (myoepithelial adenoma), (iii) Basal cell adenoma, (iv) Warthin tumour(adenolymphoma), (v) Oncocytoma (oncocytic adenoma), (vi)Canalicular adenoma, (vii) Sebaceous adenoma, (viii)Ductalpapiiloma;

(a) Inverted ductal papilloma (b) Intraductal papilloma (c) Sialadenoma papilliferum

ix) Cystadenoma (a) papillary cyst adenoma (b) Mucinous cystadenoma

B.Carcinomas:

(i) Acinic cell carcinoma, (ii) Mucoepidermoid tumour, (iii) Adenocystic carcinoma (cylindroma), (iv) Polymorphous low grade adenocarcinoma (terminal duct adenocarcinoma), (v) Epithelial-myoepithelial carcinoma, (vi) Basal cell carcinoma,(vi) Sebaceous carcinoma, (viii) Papillary Cystadenocarcinoma, (ix) Mucinous adenocarcinoma, (x) Oncocytic carcinoma, (xi) Saliva duct carcinoma, (xii) Adenocarcinoma (not otherwise specified), (xiii) Malignant Myoepithelioma (myoepithelial carcinoma), (xiv) Carcinoma in pleomorphic adenoma), (xv) Squamous cell carcinoma, (xvi) Small cell carcinoma, (xvii) Undifferentiated carcinoma, (xviii) other carcinomas

C. Non-epithelial tumours

D. Malignant lymphomas

'E. Secondary tumours

F .Unclassified tumours

G. Tumour-like lesions:

(i) Sialadenosis, (ii) Oncocytosis, (iii) Necrotizing sialometaplasia, (iv) Benign Lymphoepithelial lesion, (v) Salivary gland cysts, (vi) Chronic sclerosing sialadenitis of submandibular gland (Kuttner tumour), (vii) Cystic lymphoid hyperplasia in AIDS

7. Auto-immune disorders:

(i) Sjogren's syndrome, (ii) Benign Lymphoepithelial lesions:

(a) Godwin's (b) Mickulicz disease

8. Degenerative disorders:

(a) Hormonal: (i) Diabetes, (ii) Acromegaly, (iii) Gynecomastia, (iv) Pregnancy, (v) Menopause (b) Neurohumoral disorders (i) cardiac spasm, (ii) Gastric spasm, (iii) Bronchial asthma, (c) Disenzymatic sialosis (Hepatogenic) (d) Sialosis: (i) Metabolic, (ii) Drugs, (iii) Hormonal and, (iv) Hypoglycemic, (v) Malnutrition,

(e) Sjogren's syndrome: (i) Primary, (ii) Secondary, (iii) Aggressive, (f) Lymphoepithelial lesions: (Currently, Mickulicz disease: Sjogren's syndrome; and Mickulicz syndrome: Mostly lymphomas)

9. Age changes and oncocytosis

B. Etiological Classification:

(a) Factors influencing salivary centre:

(i) Emotions: fear, excitement, depression, (ii) Neurosis: Endogenous depression (iii) Organic disease: Brain tumour, (iv) Drugs: Atropine

(b) Factors affecting autonomic outflow pathway:

(i) Encephalitis, (ii) Brain tumour, (iii) Accident (trauma to autonomic system), (iv) Neurosurgical operation, (v) Drugs: Atropine,

(c) Factors affecting salivary gland function:

(i) Aplasia (ii) Sjogren's syndrome, (iii) Obstruction, (iv) Infection, (v) Irradiation, (vi) Excision

(d) Factors producing changes in fluid and electrolyte balance:

(i) Dehydration, (ii) Diabetes insipidus, (iii) Cardiac failure, (iv) Uremia, (v) Edema

(e) Ptyalism (Sialorrhea):

(i) Acute inflammatory conditions, e.g. Abscess, Herpes infection, Aphthae, (ii) Tooth eruption, (iii) Mental retardation, (iv) Parkinson's, (v) Schizophrenia,(vi) Mercury poisoning, (viii) Acrodynia, (ix) Rabies, (x) Familial, dysantonomia.

SPECIFIC DISEASES AND DISORDERS OF THE SALIVARY GLANDS

Developmental Abnormalities

Aplasia and Hypoplasia

The absence of salivary glands is rare although it may occur together with other developmental defects, especially malformations of the first brachial arch, which manifest with various craniofacial anomalies. Patients with salivary gland aplasia experience xerostomia and increased dental caries. Indeed, rampant dental caries in children who have no other symptoms has led to the diagnosis of congenitally missing salivary glands. Enamel hypoplasia, congenital absence of teeth, and extensive occlusal wear are other oral manifestations of salivary agenesis. Parotid gland agenesis has been reported in conjunction with several congenital conditions, including hemi facial microstomia, mandibulofacial dysostosis, cleft palate, Lacrimoauriculodentodigital syndrome, Treacher Collins syndrome, and anophthalmia. Hypoplasia of the parotid gland has been associated with Melkersson-Rosenthal syndrome. Congenital fistula formation within the ductal system has been associated with brachial cleft abnormalities, accessory parotid ducts, and diverticuli.

Aberrant salivary gland

"Aberrant" salivary glands are salivary tissues that develop at unusual anatomic sites. Aberrant salivary glands have been reported in a variety of locations, including the middle-ear cleft, external auditory canal, neck, posterior mandible, anterior mandible, pituitary, and cerebellopontine angle. These are usually incidental findings and do not require intervention. When the submandibular salivary gland sits within a depression on the lingual posterior surface of the mandible, it is referred to as Stafne's cyst. Stafne's cyst is usually located between the angle of the mandible and the first molar below the level of the inferior alveolar nerve. The gland is usually asymptomatic and appears on radiographs as a round unilocular well-circumscribed radiolucency. The characteristic location and radiographic appearance make Staphne's cyst easily recognized. Palpation of the salivary gland is possible sometimes, and sialography has been used to aid in diagnosis. Surgical intervention is recommended only in atypical situations in which the diagnosis is unclear and a tumor is suspected. Less commonly, anterior lingual submandibular salivary glands have been reported. Aberrant salivary glands occur rarely in the anterior mandible and are difficult to diagnose. They may give rise to radiolucent lesions at the apex of teeth, at extraction sites, and below and between the roots of teeth. The differential diagnosis includes the numerous unilocular radiolucent lesions of the mandible, and definitive diagnosis usually requires surgical intervention. FNA biopsy may be attempted and can yield sufficient tissue for diagnosis.

Accessory Salivary Ducts

Accessory ducts are common and do not require treatment. In a study of parotid glands by Rauch and Gorlin, half of the patients had accessory parotid ducts. The most frequent location was superior and anterior to the normal location of Stenson's duct.

Diverticuli

By definition, a diverticulum is a pouch or sac protruding from the wall of a duct. Diverticuli in the ducts of the major salivary glands often lead to pooling of saliva and recurrent sialadenitis. Diagnosis is made by sialography. Patients are encouraged to regularly milk the involved salivary gland and to promote salivary flow through the duct.

Darier's Disease

Salivary duct abnormalities have been reported in Darier's disease. Sialography of parotid glands in this condition revealed duct dilation, with periodic stricture affecting the main ducts. Symptoms of occasional obstructive sialadenitis have been reported. Progressive involvement of the salivary ducts in Darier's disease may be more common than previously reported.

Microscopically, the calcified mass exhibits concentric laminations that may surround a nidus of amorphous debris. If the associated duct also is removed, it often demonstrates squamous, oncocytic, or mucous cell metaplasia. Periductal inflammation is also evident. The ductal obstruction frequently is associated with an acute or chronic sialadenitis of the feeding gland

Treatment and Prognosis

Small sialoliths of the major glands sometimes can be treated conservatively by gentle massage of the gland in an effort to milk the stone toward the duct orifice. Sialagogues (drugs that stimulate salivary flow), moist heat, and increased fluid intake also may promote passage of the stone. Larger sialoliths usually need to be removed surgically. If significant inflammatory damage has occurred within the feeding gland, the gland may need lobe removed. Minor gland sialoliths are best treated by surgical removal, including the associated gland.

Salivary gland endoscopy is a newer method that has proven useful in the removal of some major gland sialoliths. This technique may be combined with intracorporeal lithotripsy to help fragment the stones. Extracorporeal shock wave lithotripsy also has been used successfully in Europe and Japan for the management of some patients

Inflammatory and Reactive Lesions

SIALADENITIS

Inflammation of the salivary glands (sialadenitis) can arise from various infectious and noninfectious causes. The most common viral infection is mumps, although a number of other viruses also can involve the salivary glands, including Coxsackie A, choriomeningitis, parainfluenza, and cytomegalovirus (in neonates). Most bacterial infections arise as a result of ductal obstruction or decreased salivary flow, allowing retrograde spread of bacteria throughout the ductal system. Blockage of the duct can be caused by sialolithiasis, congenital strictures, or compression by an adjacent rumor. Decreased flow can result from dehydration, debilitation, or medications that inhibit secretions. One of the more common causes of sialadenitis is recent surgery (especially abdominal surgery), after which an acute parotitis (surgical mumps) may arise because the patient has been kept without food or fluids (NPO) and has received atropine during the surgical procedure. Other medications that produce xerostomia as a side effect also can predispose patients to such an infection. Most cases of acute bacterial sialadenitis are due to Staphylococcus aureus, but they also may arise from streptococci or other organisms. Noninfectious causes of salivary inflammation include Sjogren syndrome/sarcoidosis, radiation therapy, and various allergens.

Clinical and Radiographic Features

Acute bacterial sialadenitis is most common in the parotid gland and is bilateral in 10% to 25% of cases. The affected gland is swollen and painful, and the overlying skin maybe erythematous. An associated low-grade fever may be present, as well as trismus. A purulent discharge often is observed from the duct orifice when the gland is massaged.

Recurrent or persistent ductal obstruction (most commonly caused by sialoliths can lead to a chronic sialadenitis. Periodic swelling and pain occur within the affected gland, usually developing at mealtime when salivary flow is stimulated. Sialography often demonstrates sialectasia (ductal dilatation) proximal to the area of obstruction. In the submandibular gland, persistent enlargement may occur (Kuttner tumor), which is difficult to distinguish from a true neoplasm. Chronic sialadenitis also can occur in the minor glands, possibly as a result of blockage of ductal flow or local trauma.

Subacute necrotizing sialadenitis is a recently recognized form of salivary inflammation that occurs most commonly in teenagers and young adults. The lesion usually involves the minor salivary glands of the hard or soft palate, presenting as a painful nodule that is covered by intact, erythematous mucosa. Unlike necrotizing sialometaplasia, the lesion does not ulcerate or slough necrotic tissue. An infectious or allergic cause has been hypothesized.

Histopathologic Features

In patients with acute sialadenitis, accumulation of neutrophils is observed within the ductal system and acini. Chronic sialadenitis is characterized by scattered or patchy infiltration of the salivary parenchyma by lymphocytes and plasma cells. Atrophy of the acini is common, as is ductal dilatation. If associated fibrosis is present, the term chronic sclerosing sialadenitis is used. Subacute necrotizing sialadenitis is characterized by a heavy mixed inflammatory infiltrate consisting of neutrophils, lymphocytes, histiocytes, and eosinophils. There is loss of most of the acinar cells, and many of the remaining ones exhibit necrosis. The ducts tend to atrophic and do not show hyperplasia or squamous metaplasia.

Treatment and Prognosis

The treatment of acute sialadenitis includes appropriate antibiotic therapy and rehydration of the patient to stimulate salivary flow. Surgical drainage may be needed if there is abscess formation. Although this regimen is usually sufficient, a 20% to 50% mortality rate has beer reported in debilitated patients because of the spread of the infection and sepsis.

The management of chronic sialadenitis depends on the severity and duration of the condition. Early cases that develop secondary to ductal blockage may respond to removal of the sialolith or other obstruction. If sialectasia is present, the dilated ducts can lead to stasis of secretions and predispose the gland to further sialolith formation. If sufficient inflammatory destruction of the salivary tissue has occurred, surgical removal of the affected gland may be necessary.

Subacute necrotizing sialadenitis is a self-limiting condition that usually resolves within 2 weeks of diagnosis without treatment.

BACTERIAL SIALADENITIS

Etiology

Bacterial infections of the salivary glands are most commonly seen in patients with reduced salivary gland function .This condition was formerly referred to as "surgical parotitis" because post surgery patients often experienced gland enlargement from ascending bacterial infections. This was thought to relate to the markedly decreased salivary flow during anesthesia, often as the result of administered anticholinergic drugs and relative dehydration due to restricted fluids. With the administration of prophylactic antibiotics and routine perioperative hydration, this condition now occurs much less frequently. Raad and colleagues reported only three instances in 300,000 cases occurring postoperatively.

Today, the majority of bacterial infections occur in patients with disease- or medication-induced salivary gland hypo function. The reduction of salivary flow results in diminished mechanical flushing, which allows bacteria to colonize the oral cavity and then to invade the salivary duct and cause acute bacterial infection. Studies have shown that poor oral hygiene contributes to salivary gland bacterial infections. The geriatric population is particularly susceptible to bacterial sialadenitis due to the frequent combination of medication-induced xerostomia and poor oral hygiene. The habit of fecal ingestion also has been associated with sialadenitis. Although sialoliths occur more frequently in the submandibular glands, bacterial sialadenitis occurs more frequently in the parotid glands. It is theorized that the submandibular glands may be protected by the high level of mucin in the saliva, which has potent antimicrobial activity. Anatomy may also play a protective role; tongue movements tend to clear the floor of the mouth and protect Wharton's duct. In contrast, the orifice of Stenson's duct is located adjacent to the molars, where heavy bacterial colonization occurs. Other possible causes include trauma to the duct system and hematogerious spread of infection from other areas. The most commonly isolated organisms in parotitis are penicillin-resistant Staphylococcus aureus, Streptococcus viridians, and Streptococcus pneumonias. It is of interest to note the marked reduction in the overall incidence of acute parotitis after the introduction of antibiotic preparations. As resistant strains of bacteria have appeared, the prevalence of acute parotitis has increased.

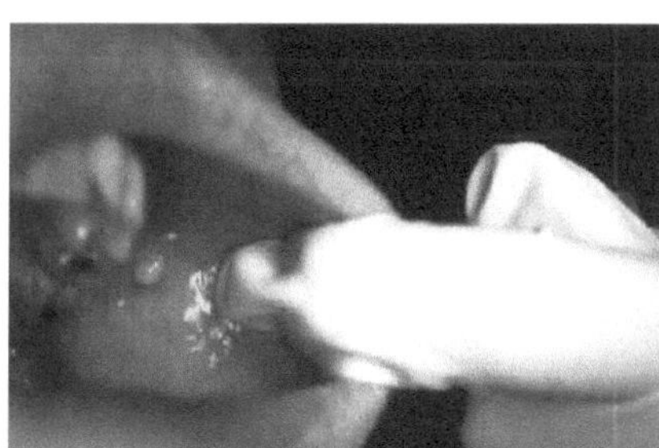

Clinical Presentation

Patients usually present with a sudden onset of unilateral or bilateral salivary gland enlargement. Approximately 20% of the cases present as bilateral infections. The involved gland is painful, indurated, and tender to palpation. The overlying skin may be erythematous.

. Laboratory studies disclose an elevated erythrocyte sedimentation rate (ESR) and leukocytosis, often with a characteristic shift to the left, indicating acute infection. The involved gland is extremely tender, with the patient often demonstrating guarding during examination. Trismus is often noted, and purulence at the duct orifice may be produced by gentle pressure on the involved gland or duct. If the infection is not eliminated early, suppuration may extend beyond the limiting capsule of the parotid gland. Extension into surrounding tissues along fascial planes in the neck or extension posteriorly into the external auditory canal may follow. A purulent discharge may be expressed from the duct orifice, and samples of this exudate should be cultured for aerobes and anaerobes. A second specimen should be sent for testing with Gram's stain. The most commonly cultured organisms include coagulase- positive Staphylococcus aureus, Streptococcus viridans, Streptococcus pneumoniae, Escherichia coli, and Haemophilus influenzae. Institutionalized individuals are particularly susceptible to infections caused by methicillin-resistant Staphylococcus aureus. Due to the dense capsule surrounding the salivary glands, it is difficult to determine, based on physical examination alone, whether an abscess has formed. Ultrasonography or CT is recommended for visualizing possible cystic areas.

Treatment and Prognosis

Management of bacterial sialadenitis is directed at elimination of the causative organism coupled with rehydration of the patient and drainage of purulence, if present. Culture and sensitivity testing of the exudate at the orifice of the duct is the first step in antibiotic management. After a culture is obtained, all patients should empirically be placed on a regimen of a penicillinase-resistant antibiotic such as semisynthetic penicillin. Along with rehydration and attempts at establishing and encouraging salivary flow, moist compresses, analgesics, and rest are in order. Medications containing parasympathomimetic agents, which reduce salivary flow, should be reduced or eliminated. If a purulent discharge is present, empiric intravenous administration of a penicillinase- resistant antistaphylococcal antibiotic is indicated. Patients should be instructed to "milk" the involved gland several times throughout the day. Increased hydration and improved oral hygiene are required. With these measures, significant improvement should be noted within 24 to 48 hours. If this does not occur, then incision and drainage should be considered. The mortality rate for bacterial sialadenitis was once high, but the availability of a selection of broad-spectrum antibiotics has eliminated mortality in noncritically ill patients. As salivary gland enlargement may be nonbacterial in origin, such as in virally induced swelling or in Sjögren's syndrome, antibiotics should not be started routinely unless bacterial infection is clinically obvious.

A biopsy and retrograde sialography should be avoided. The former may cause sinus tract formation, and the latter may allow infection to proceed beyond the boundaries of the gland into surrounding soft tissues. With prompt and effective treatment, recurrence is generally avoided. In cases of recurrent parotitis, considerable destructive glandular changes can be seen.

In the so-called juvenile variant of parotitis, intermittent unilateral or bilateral painful swelling is accompanied by fever and malaise. The initial attack usually occurs in individuals between ages 2 and 6 years, with numerous recurrences thereafter. Rarely a neonatal form of suppurative parotitis may develop, with S. aureus being the most common causative pathogen. Gross destruction of the parenchymal and ductal elements may be noted on sialographic examination. Absence of secretory acinar components and a damaged ductal system with numerous punctate globular spaces may be seen. Spontaneous regeneration of parotid salivary tissue has been reported in this condition.

Viral Diseases

Viruses have been associated with acute nonsuppurative salivary gland enlargement. This section focuses on the viruses responsible for the majority of cases of virally induced salivary gland enlargement: Paramyxovirus, Cytomegalovirus (CMV), HIV, and hepatitis C virus (HCV). Echoviruses, Epstein-Barr virus, parainfluenza virus, and choriomeningitis virus infections have been linked to occasional reports of nonsuppurative salivary gland enlargement.

MUMPS (EPIDEMIC PAROTITIS)

Mumps is an infectious, acute viral sialadenitis affecting primarily the parotid glands. Considered the most common of all salivary gland diseases before the advent of routine immunization, it has a year-round endemic pattern, although seasonal peaks are noted in the late winter and spring months.

Etiology and Pathogenesis

The causative agent of mumps is a Paramyxovirus. A 2 to 3-week incubation period precedes clinical symptoms. Transmission is by direct contact with salivary droplets. The United States and Canada have recommended the mumps vaccine since the 1970s and monitor vaccinations at school admission. An attenuated live vaccine is available and is indicated for immunization against mumps in children aged 12 months or older. The incidence of mumps in developed countries has significantly decreased; in the United States, 906 cases were reported in 1995. The Centers for Disease Control and Prevention (CDC) published modifications to the Recommended Childhood Immunization Schedule in 1998. The CDC currently recommends an initial vaccination at 12 to 18 months of age and a second dose at 4 to 6 years of age. Mumps virus vaccine is not recommended for severely immunocompromised children because the protective immune response often does not develop, and risk of complications exists. There has been speculation that the Measles-Mumps-Rubella (MMR) Vaccine might be linked to autism and inflammatory bowel disease, which raised parental concern. Although epidemiologic studies demonstrate no evidence for a causal association between MMR administration and these conditions, many parents have refused vaccination for their children. This raises public health concerns as it results in a susceptible population and the possibility of the re-emergence of mumps in the United States. International travelers who have not had mumps or been vaccinated can import the virus. In 1997, an outbreak of mumps among adults (ages 17 to 40 years) attending "rare" parties was reported in Vancouver, British Columbia. Therefore, this infection must be considered in cases of acute nonsuppurative salivary gland inflammation in unvaccinated patients who have not had mumps.

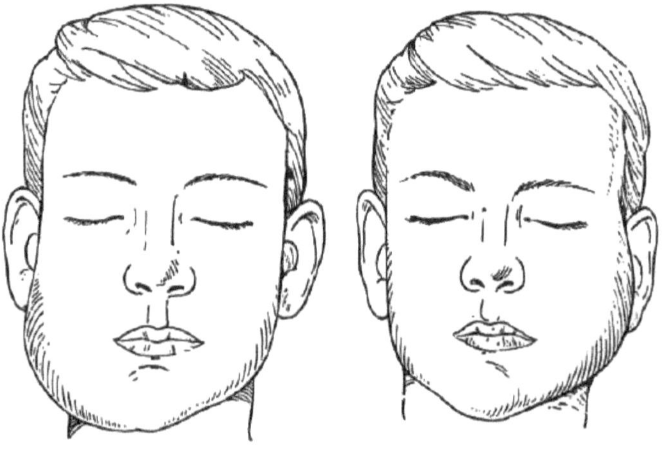

Clinical Presentation

The disease affects males and females equally, especially young adults and children. Ordinarily, mumps occurs in children between the ages of 4 and 6 years. The diagnosis of mumps in adults can be more difficult. The incubation period is 2 to 3 weeks; this is followed by salivary gland inflammation and enlargement, preauricular pain, fever, malaise, headache, and myalgia. The majority of cases involve the parotid glands, but 10% of the cases involve the submandibular glands alone. The skin over the involved glands is edematous. The salivary gland enlargement is sudden and painful to palpation. The salivary gland ducts are inflammed but without purulent discharge. If partial duct obstruction occurs, the patient may experience pain when eating. One gland can become symptomatic 24 to 48 hours before another gland does so. Swelling is usually bilateral and lasts approximately 7 days The diagnosis is made by the demonstration of antibodies to the mumps S and V antigens and to the hemagglutination antigen. Serum amylase levels may be elevated. Potentially serious complications (orchitis or oophoritis) can occur in adults. Mumps is a systemic infection, as evidenced by the widespread involvement of glandular and other tissues in the body, including the liver, pancreas, kidney, and nervous system. Complications of mumps include mild meningitis and encephalitis. Deafness, myocarditis, thyroiditis, pancreatitis, and oophoritis occur less frequently .Males can experience epididymitis and orchitis, resulting in testicular atrophy and infertility if the disease occurs in adolescence or later.

Treatment and Prognosis

Treatment is symptomatic and includes bed rest. Analgesics are prescribed, and in severe cases corticosteroids may be used. Complete recovery is generally the rule, although fatalities have been associated with viral encephalitis, myocarditis, and nephritis. Nerve deafness and bilateral testicular atrophy have been noted but are uncommon.

Prevention of the disease is now possible using a live attenuated vaccine that induces a non communicable, sub clinical infection. Antibody conversion occurs in approximately 90% of susceptible individuals, and immunity is life long. Although mumps is the most common form of viral sialadenitis, it is important to note that parotitis may also be caused by other viral agents, including coxsackie A virus, echovirus, choriomeningitis virus, cytomegalovirus, and parainfluenza virus types 1 and 2.

CYTOMEGALOVIRUS INFECTION

Cytomegalovirus infection of salivary glands, or so-called cytomegalic inclusion disease, is a rare condition that affects neonates as a result of transplacental infection. Systemic disease may cause debilitation, developmental retardation, and premature birth.

When encountered in adults who are inununo-suppressed (e.g., human immunodeficiency virus [HIV] infection, organ transplants), infection may cause fever, salivary gland enlargement, hepatosplenomegaly, pneumonitis, and lymphocytosis. Retinitis can be a serious complication of this infection. Adults who are not immunosuppressed may also be infected with cytomegalovirus, as evidenced by demonstration of antibodies in serum. Symptomatology may be nonexistent, or there may be slight to debilitating fever and malaise. The significance of cytomegalovirus infections in this population is poorly understood.

Etiology

Human CMV is a beta herpes virus that infects only humans. CMV may remain latent after initial exposure and infection. Although its reactivation can occur in healthy individuals without clinical illness, reactivation in immunocompromised individuals can be life threatening. CMV can be cultured from blood, saliva, feces, respiratory secretions, urine, and other body fluids. A large percentage of healthy adults have serum antibodies to the virus. CMV is the major cause of non-Epstein-Barr virus infectious mononucleosis in the general population. Horizontal transmission can occur through blood transfusion, allograft transplants, and sexual contact .Particularly high rates of seropositivity are found in homosexual males, intravenous drug users, prostitutes, and individuals who have undergone multiple transfusions.

Transmission from children to adults or between children is more common through fomites, urine, and respiratory secretions. Transplacental spread of CMV may result in congenital infection and malformations. Perinatal infection occurs in 3% of all live births and is thought to be due to transmission from breast milk, saliva, fomites, or urine. Infection in newborns and young children can be fatal.

Clinical Presentation

CMV mononucleosis often occurs in the young adult population and presents as an acute febrile illness that includes salivary gland enlargement. Diagnosis is based on an elevated titer of antibody to CMV, and the prognosis for healthy adults is excellent. There is one report (by Guntinas-Lichius and colleagues) of acute severe CMV sialadenititis in a 57-year-old immunocompetent male who required hospitalization for 30 days. It is important to detect CMV infections in pregnant women. Transplacental transmission of CMV can result in prematurity, low birth weight, and various congenital malformations. Infected newborns and young children suffer from hepatitis, myocarditis, hematologic abnormalities, pneumonitis, and nervous system damage. The infection is often fatal; those children who do survive frequently experience permanent nerve damage resulting in mental retardation and seizure disorders. Infection in adults can occur by reactivation of the latent virus or by primary infection. An impaired immune system allows the virus to replicate and allows disseminated infection to occur. Patients taking immunosuppressive medications and patients with hematologic abnormalities or HIV infection are susceptible to severe CMV infections. In fact, CMV is considered a clinical marker for acquired immunodeficiency syndrome (AIDS). The CDC's surveillance case definition for AIDS includes CMV infection of the salivary glands that lasts longer than 1 month in adult patients. CMV infection also is strongly associated with an increased incidence of fungal and bacterial infections, particularly from gram-negative organisms. The advent of highly active antiretroviral therapy (HAART) for treating HIV infection has resulted in a decline of CMV end-organ damage. Deayton and colleagues reported that HAART (including a protease inhibitor) suppresses CMV viremia in HIV-infected patients who are not receiving specific anti-CMV therapy. There are no published reports addressing the incidence of CMV-related salivary gland pathology in HIV-infected patients since the widespread adoption of HAART.

The diagnosis of CMV infection may be difficult because of the issues of viral latency in many individuals, past virus infection versus acute clinical disease, and reactivation. The classic method for detection is histologic examination of infected tissue. CMV-infected tissue contains large atypical cells with inclusion bodies. These cells can be two times the normal size and have eccentrically placed nuclei, resulting in an "owl-like" appearance. Tissue necrosis and nonspecific inflammation may also be seen histologically. Current methods for diagnosis include culture, antigen detection, and CMV deoxyribonucleic acid (DNA) detection.

Diagnosis of primary infection in an immunocompetent patient uses a combination of immunoglobulin M (IgM) anti- CMV antibody seropositivity, IgG seroconversion, and viral culture. Antibodies to CMV are less useful diagnostically in immunocompromised individuals. Anti-CMV antibodies can be falsely negative in transplantation patients and falsely positive in patients with autoimmune disease. The virus can be detected directly in body fluids or tissue by culture, antigen assay, or CMV DNA assay. The presence of IgG antibodies against CMV is used to detect past CMV infection in immunocompetent patients who are being screened for blood or organ donation.

Treatment

Immunocompetent patients are treated symptomatically. Immunocompromised patients require aggressive management and may be treated with intravenous gancyclovir, foscarnet, or cidofovir. Alive attenuated vaccine is in clinical trials and has demonstrated partial protection in seronegative women exposed to seropositive infants and in seronegative kidney transplant recipients who received organs from seropositive donors. It is speculated that vaccineinduced immunity will be less effective against sexually transmitted CMV infection, in which re-infection with wild virus strains occurs.

HIV INFECTION

Etiology

Neoplastic and non-neoplastic salivary gland lesions occur with increased frequency in HIV-infected patients. Clinicians should consider AIDS-related tumors such as Kaposi's sarcoma and lymphoma. A Sjögren's syndrome– like phenomenon is also seen in HIV-infected patients. A variety of terms have been used to describe this condition; "HIV salivary gland disease" (HIV-SGD) is the preferred term. HIV-SGD describes xerostomia and benign (unilateral or bilateral) salivary gland enlargement in HIVpositive patients. The prevalence of HIV-SGD is ≈1.0% in adult HIV-infected patients but has been reported to be as high as 19% in pediatric patients. Adult African Americans experience lesions more frequently than Caucasians based on data in the US. Homosexual persons and intravenous drug users experience gland enlargement more frequently than patients infected by other routes of transmission. The etiology of HIV-SGD is not understood, but the reactivation of a latent virus has been hypothesized. Changes in the incidence of parotid hypertrophy since the advent of HAART have not been reported. HIV-SGD is associated with a cluster designation 8 (CD8) cell lymphocytosis of the salivary glands and with the diffuse infiltrative lymphocytosis syndrome (DILS). In this condition, lymphocytic infiltration is found in the salivary glands, lungs, gastrointestinal tract, and liver. Modest changes in salivary function without enlargement have also been reported. Greenberg and colleagues studied two groups of HIV-infected patients: one group with xerostomia and one group without xerostomia. Both groups were evaluated for the presence of CMV in saliva, blood, labial minor salivary glands, and peripheral blood mononuclear cells.115 Xerostomia and reduced salivary flow were associated with the presence of CMV. These results suggest a potential link between CMV in saliva and salivary gland dysfunction in HIV-infected patients.

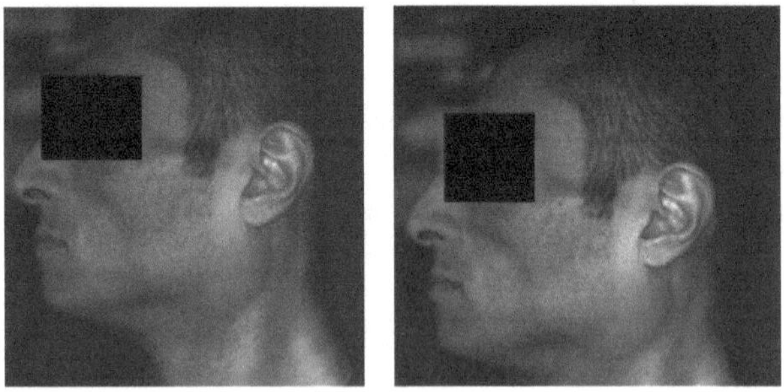

Clinical Manifestations

The most notable symptom of HIVSGD is salivary gland swelling, which may or may not be accompanied by xerostomia. The parotid glands are involved in 98% of reported cases, and 60% of patients have bilateral enlargement. HIV SGD frequently resembles Sjögren's syndrome and must be distinguished from this disorder by appropriate evaluation including salivary flow rates, ophthalmologic evaluation (with assessments of lacrimal function and the tear film), and autoimmune serologies. Ten percent of HIV-infected patients have a reduced lacrimal flow. Salivary flow rates may be reduced and salivary immunoglobulin A (IgA) may be elevated both in patients with Sjögren's syndrome and in patients with HIV-SGD. Peripheral blood changes can resemble the changes seen in cases of Sjögren's syndrome and include hypergammaglobulinemia, circulating immune complexes, and rheumatoid factors. However, anti-SS-A and anti-SS-B autoantibodies are usually negative in the HIV-SGD population. A minor salivary gland biopsy may be indicated, and histologic findings resemble changes seen in cases of Sjögren's syndrome (including focal mononuclear cell infiltration) with routine tissue examination. Using immunohistochemical stains to differentiate the infiltrating cells, one finds a preponderance of CD8-positive (+) cells in HIV-SGD, as compared to the CD4+ infiltrates that predominate in Sjögren's syndrome.

If there is involvement of the major salivary glands, they can be imaged with ultrasonography, CT, or MRI. Multiple cystic masses are characteristic of HIV-associated benign lymphoepithelial hypertrophy. With persistent enlargement of a major gland, a biopsy of the affected tissue may be necessary to exclude neoplasia. Of particular concern are lymphoma and Kaposi's sarcoma, both of which have been reported in the salivary glands of HIV-infected individuals. A biopsy specimen from an HIV-SGD–involved major gland demonstrates hyperplastic lymph nodes, lymphocytic infiltates, and cystic cavities.

When assessing the HIV infected patient who has salivary complaints, it is important to consider that this patient group also frequently experiences medication-induced xerostomia. When salivary gland enlargement is present, bacterial infection should also be considered.

Treatment

Treatment for HIVSGD is primarily symptomatic. Xerostomia may be relieved by sipping water, using saliva substitutes, chewing sugar-free gum, or sucking sugar-free candy. Topical fluoride is suggested for control of caries. Benign parotid enlargement is an esthetic concern for some patients, and surgery has been performed for cosmetic reasons. Treatment of the enlargement with external radiation therapy has also been attempted, but only 1 of 12 HIV-infected patients with parotid hypertrophy who were treated with 8 to 10 Gy of radiotherapy to the affected gland had a reduction in gland size. In 68% of patients, 24 Gy delivered in 1.5 Gy doses was effective, and 70% of those cases had a clinical benefit lasting 2 years. The potential for radiation-induced malignancy does exist, and clinicians must schedule regular follow-up visits to monitor for malignant changes. Radiation therapy also may increase the degree of xerostomia. It is speculated that systemic anti-HIV treatment may augment radiation therapy. However, antiretroviral treatments alone have shown minimal effects on enlarged parotid glands. Two other methods of treatment include the aspiration of cysts and tetracycline sclerosis. The injection of a tetracycline solution into cystic areas will sometimes induce an inflammatory reaction and eventual sclerosis. Formal studies with long-term follow-up have not been reported for these methods.

HEPATITIS C VIRUS INFECTION

Etiology

Viruses have been considered potential triggers of autoimmune diseases for many years. Retroviruses are known to infect cells of the immune system and to disrupt immunoregulation. Sicca symptoms mimicking Sjögren's syndrome have been described in diseases caused by retroviruses (see discussion of HIV-SGD, above).Hepatitis C virus (HCV) DNA has been detected in the saliva of patients with chronic hepatitis C infection, and it has been demonstrated that the saliva of HCV carriers is infective. A number of reports from European centers have suggested an association between HCV and Sjögren's syndrome. Subsequent investigations reported conflicting results. King and colleagues examined 48 Sjögren's syndrome patients and reported them negative for HCV. Marrone and colleagues found that none of their 100 well-characterized Sjögren's syndrome patients had evidence of acute or chronic HCV infection. In contrast, Pawlotsky and colleagues looked at a series of HCV-infected patients and found that 14% had a salivary gland pathology that resembled Sjögren's syndrome. These differences in results may be due to population variability and differing case definitions. The prevalence of asymptomatic HCV infection is higher in Europe than in the United States. Also, different authors have used less stringent diagnostic criteria for Sjögren's syndrome. When stringent diagnostic criteria have been applied and studies have been done in populations with relatively low endemic HCV infection, an increase of HCV infection in Sjögren's syndrome has not been found .However, the potential relationship between HCV and autoimmune disease remains an area of continuing debate. Although a causal relationship between autoimmune disease and HCV is unlikely, salivary gland pathology can be noted in HCV-infected patients. Haddad and colleagues reported that

16 of 28 HCV-infected patients in their study had sialadenitis resembling Sjögren's syndrome. Scott and colleagues performed biopsies of labial minor salivary glands in HCV-infected patients and found lymphoid aggregates, duct ectasia, lymphocytic infiltrates, and acinar depletion. Pirisi and colleagues reported that specimens from lip biopsies from 17 of 22 HCV-positive patients demonstrated inflammatory changes similar to those seen in patients with Sjögren's syndrome. The inflammation seen in the HCV-infected population was described as mild compared to that seen in Sjögren's syndrome patients.

Clinical Manifestations

HCV infection has many extra hepatic manifestations, including salivary gland enlargement. Patients may report xerostomia along with chronic major salivary gland enlargement. Both Scott and colleagues and Haddad and colleagues reported that females with chronic HCV infection had a greater tendency for sialadenitis. Clinical manifestations and salivary histologic lesions generally are significantly milder in patients with chronic HCV infection than in patients with Sjögren's syndrome. It is worth noting that HCV-infected patients do not commonly experience dry eyes along with xerostomia. The diagnosis of HCV infection is made by the detection of anti-HCV antibodies and HCV DNA

Treatment

Hepatitis-associated sialadenitis is treated symptomatically.

ALLERGIC SIALADENITIS

Enlargement of the salivary glands has been associated with exposure to various pharmaceutical agents and allergens. Cases that are without rash or other signs of allergy have been reported. The characteristic feature of such an allergic reaction is acute salivary gland enlargement, often accompanied by itching over the gland. It is unclear whether all of the reported cases are true allergic reactions or some represent secondary infections resulting from medications that reduced salivary flow. Compounds have salivary gland enlargement as a potential side effect include phenobarbital, phenothiazine, ethambutol, sulfisoxazole, iodine compounds, isoproterenol, and heavy metals. The diagnosis of allergic reaction should be made judiciously, especially when salivary gland enlargement is not accompanied by other signs of an allergic reaction. The possibility of infection or autoimmune disease should be considered.

Allergic sialadenitis is self-limiting. Avoiding the allergen, maintaining hydration, and monitoring for secondary infection are recommended

RADIATION-INDUCED PATHOLOGY

Effects of External-Beam Radiation

External-beam radiation is standard treatment for head and neck tumors, and the salivary glands are often within the field of radiation. Doses of $\geq$ 50 Gy will result in permanent salivary gland damage and symptoms of oral dryness. The exact mechanism of the destruction of salivary gland tissue by radiation is not fully understood.

Clinical Presentation

Radiotherapy is usually delivered in fractionated doses 5 days per week for 6 to 8 weeks. Acute effects on salivary function can be recognized within a week of beginning treatments at doses of approximately 2 Gy daily and patients will often voice complaints of oral dryness by the end of the second week .Mucositis is a very common consequence of treatment and can become severe enough to alter the radiation therapy regimen. If permanent salivary dysfunction develops, patients are at risk of the full range of associated oral complications. Typically, at doses > 50 Gy, salivary dysfunction is severe and permanent. Difficulty in speaking, dysphagia, and increased dental caries are common complaints that dramatically affect the quality of life for patients with radiation-induced salivary gland dysfunction. Saliva is minimal, and the saliva that is present tends to be thick and ropy.

"Radiation caries" is the term commonly used to describe these patients' rapidly advancing caries, which characteristically occur at the incisal or cervical aspect of the teeth and wrap around the teeth in an "apple core" fashion. In spite of meticulous oral hygiene, the caries rate is often difficult to control and poses a challenge to even the experienced restorative dentist. This patient population is susceptible to other oral complications, including candidiasis and sialadenitis. Clinicians should always be aware of the risk of osteonecrosis and the increased incidence of salivary gland neoplasms in postradiation patients. Osteonecrosis is a lifelong risk due to the decreased vascularity following the exposure of bone to radiation.

There is also an increased incidence of second primary tumors involving the radiated tissues.

Treatment

Radiation planning is key to the effective preservation of salivary gland tissue. Eisbrush and colleagues reported that when three-dimensional comformal radiation therapy was used in patients receiving bilateral head and neck radiation with the goal of limiting salivary exposure, 50% of salivary gland function was preserved. Tumor control and complications are still being assessed, but this technique appears to offer real benefit. In addition to improvements in the planning and delivery of radiation therapy, radioprotective agents may help limit radiation therapy–induced salivary gland damage. Starting in the 1970s, studies have investigated the radioprotective properties of amifostine; however, not until 1999 was amifostine approved as a radioprotective agent by the Food and Drug Administration. This agent is useful for the preservation of salivary function and for the reduction of dry mouth in patients undergoing radiation treatment for head and neck cancer when the radiation port includes a substantial portion of the parotid glands. The proposed mechanism of action involves the scavenging of free oxygen radicals. Following administration, amifostine is dephosphorylated in the circulation by alkaline phosphatase to a pharmacologically active free thiol metabolite. The thiol metabolite scavenges free oxygen species generated by radiation .Normal tissue is more vascular than the tumor and has higher capillary levels of alkaline phosphatase. Therefore, the concentration of the active thiol metabolite is higher in normal tissue and thus will protect the normal tissue but not the cancer. Amifostine is administered intravenously 15 to 30 minutes prior to each fractionated radiation treatment. Major side effects include hypotension, hypocalemia, nausea, and vomiting. Reversible episodes of loss of consciousness and rare incidences of seizures have been reported. This drug should be used with close supervision in patients taking hypertension medications. Its safety for patients with cardiovascular disease or cerebrovascular conditions has not been studied.

Since patients undergoing radiation therapy have reduced salivary flow, they are susceptible to oral fungal and bacterial infections. Candidal infections can be difficult to treat and resistant to therapy. Due to the increased risk of caries, antifungal agents should be free of sugar. Vaginal clotrimazole troches and dissolved nystatin powder may be used orally as sugar-free antifungal agents. Since xerostomic patients may have too little saliva to dissolve troches, antifungal oral rinses are preferred. Daily prescription-strength topical fluoride (which can be brushed on or administered in trays) is recommended to help control caries. Symptomatic treatment for post radiation patients is discussed in detail later in this chapter, in the section on the treatment of xerostomia. Alternative medicine is gaining popularity in Western culture and medical curricula. Studies investigating acupuncture treatment for radiation-induced xerostomia have reported varying results. Chi gong and herbal medications are alternative therapies that are reported to increase salivary flow. More controlled trials of these therapeutic modalities are needed

Effects of Internal Radiation Therapy

Etiology

Disseminated thyroid cancer (DTC) is treated by the removal of the thyroid gland. To ensure that all remnants of thyroid tissue are destroyed, patients are given radioactive iodine 131 (131I) after surgery. Radioactive iodine is taken up not only by thyroid tissue but also by the oncocytes in salivary gland tissue. Radioactive iodine can cause permanent salivary gland damage and fibrosis resulting in salivary gland hypo function. Mandel and colleagues recently reported changes in saliva composition following 131I therapy. It is believed that salivary gland damage is related to the dose of 131I administered.

Clinical Presentation

Patients with DTC treated with131I may experience xerostomia and decreased salivary gland function. However, 131I treatment is less caustic than external-beam radiation therapy and generally causes less destruction to the salivary glands.

Treatment

Following administration of 131I, patients should suck on lemon drops or chew gum to stimulate salivary flow. This will aid in clearing the radioactive iodine from the salivary glands and will potentially decrease salivary gland damage. Patients with 131I-induced salivary gland hypo function should be treated with the same measures as patients who have salivary gland damage from other causes.

CHEILITIS GLANDULARIS

Cheilitis glandularis is a rare inflammatory condition of the minor salivary glands. The cause is uncertain, although several etiologic factors have been suggested, including actinic damage, tobacco, syphilis, poor hygiene, and heredity.

Clinical Features

Cheilitis glandularis characteristically occurs on the lower lip, although there are also purported cases involving the upper lip and palate. Affected individuals experience swelling and eversion of the lower lip as a result of hypertrophy and inflammation of the glands . The openings of the minor salivary ducts are inflamed and dilated, and pressure on the glands may produce mucopurulent secretions from the ductal openings. The condition most often has been reported in middle-aged and older men, although cases also have been described in women and children. However, some of the childhood cases may represent other entities, such as exfoliative cheilitis.

Historically, cheilitis glandularis has been classified into three types, based on the severity of the disease:

1. Simple
2. Superficial suppurative (Baelz's disease)
3. Deep suppurative (cheilitis glandularis apostematosal)

The latter two types represent progressive stages of the disease with bacterial involvement and are characterized by increasing inflammation, suppuration, ulceration, and swelling of the lip.

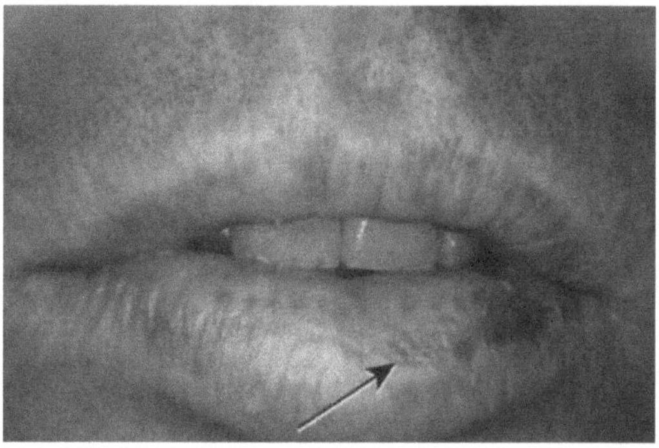

Histopathologic Features

The microscopic findings of cheilitis glandularis arc not specific and usually consist of chronic sialadenitis and ductal dilatation. Concomitant dysplastic changes may be observed in the overlying surface epithelium in some cases.

Treatment and Prognosis

The treatment of choice for most cases of persistent cheilitis glandularis associated with acinic damage is vermilionectomy (lip shave), which usually produces a satisfactory cosmetic result. A significant percentage of cases (18% to 35%) have been associated with the development of squamous cell carcinoma of the overlying epithelium of the lip. Because acinic damage has been implicated in many cases of cheilitis glandularis, it is likely that this same solar radiation is responsible for the malignant degeneration.

ADENOMATOID HYPERPLASIA OF THE MINOR SALIVARY GLANDS

Adenomatoid hyperplasia is a non neoplastic enlargement of the minor salivary glands of the hard palate.

Clinical Features

Adenomatoid hyperplasia is a rare lesion of the minor salivary glands characterized by localized swelling that mimics a neoplasm. This pseudotumor most often occurs on the hard or soft palate, although it also has been reported in other oral minor salivary gland sites. The pathogenesis of adenomatoid hyperplasia is uncertain, but it has been speculated that local trauma may play a role. It is most common in the fourth to sixth decades of life. Most examples present as sessile, painless masses that may be soft or firm to palpation. They usually are normal in color, although a few lesions are red or bluish.

Histopathologic Features

Microscopic examination demonstrates lobular aggregates of relatively normal-appearing mucous acini that are greater in number than normally would be found in the area. These glands also sometimes appear to be increased in size. In some instances, the glands arc situated close to the mucosal surface. Chronic inflammation occasionally is seen, but it usually is mild and localized in nature.

Differential Diagnosis

A clinical differential diagnosis would include salivary neoplasms, lymphoma, and extension of nasopharyngeal or sinonasal disease into the oral cavity. Periapical inflammatory disease should be excluded.

Treatment and Prognosis

Because the clinical presentation of adenomatoid hyperplasia mimics a tumor, biopsy is necessary to establish the diagnosis. Once the diagnosis has been established, no further treatment is indicated and the lesion should not recur.

SIALADENOSIS (SIALOSIS)

Sialadenosis is an unusual noninflammatory disorder characterized by salivary gland enlargement, particularly involving the parotid glands. The condition frequently is associated with an underlying systemic problem, which may be endocrine, nutritional, or neurogenic in origin. The best known of these conditions include diabetes mellitus, general malnutrition, alcoholism, and bulimia.

These conditions are believed to result in dysregulation of the autonomic innervation of the salivary acini, causing an aberrant intracellular secretory cycle. This leads to excessive accumulation of secretory granules, with marked enlargement of the acinar cells.

Conditions Associated With Sialadenosis

A. ENDOCRINE

Diabetes mellitus

* Diabetes insipidus
* Acromegaly
* Hypothyroidisrn
* Pregnancy

B. NUTRITIONAL

* General malnutrition
* Alcoholism
* Anorexia nervosa
* Bulimia

C. NEUROCENIC MEDICATIONS

* Antihypertensive drugs
* Psychotropic drugs
* Sympathomimetic drugs used for treating asthma

Alcoholic cirrhosis or chronic alcoholism and asymptomatic enlargement of the parotid glands occur in 30% to 80% of patients. Salivary gland enlargement has been attributed to chronic protein deficiency. Comparable parotid gland enlargement in individuals with cirrhosis due to other causes apparently does not occur. Nutritional or protein deprivation may also lead to a similar salivary gland enlargement.

In diabetes mellitus, reduced flow rates have been reported in addition to bilateral parotid gland enlargement. The mechanism of acinar hypertrophy in this condition is unknown. Reduced flow rates from the parotid and other major salivary glands may lead to an increased risk of bacterial sialadenitis.

In cases of type I hyperlipoproteinemia a sicca-like syndrome has been described. This is characterized primarily by parotid enlargement with mild oral or ocular sicca symptoms; it is generally attributed to the presence of fatly replacement of functional salivary gland parenchyma.

Another endocrine-related salivary gland enlargement may be noted in acromegaly. This may merely be a reflection of a generalized organomegaly encountered in this endocrine-mediated disturbance. Apparent parotid enlargement {acinar hypertrophy) and increased levels of parotid flow have also been noted in patients having chronic relapsing pancreatitis.

Clinical and Radiographic Features

Sialadenosis usually appears as a slowly evolving swelling of the parotid glands, which may or may not be painful. The condition is usually bilateral, but it also can be unilateral. In some patients, the submandibular glands can be involved. Decreased salivary secretion may occur. Sialography demonstrates a "leafless tree" pattern, which is thought to be caused by compression of the finer ducts by hyperirophic acinar cells.

Histopathologic Features

Microscopic examination reveals hypertrophy of the acinar cells, sometimes two to three times greater than normal size. The nuclei are displaced to the cell base, and the cytoplasm is engorged with zymogen granules. Incases associated with longstanding diabetes or alcoholism, there may be acinar atrophy and fatty infiltration. Significant inflammation is not observed.

Treatment and Prognosis

The clinical management of sialadenosis is often unsatisfactory because it is closely related to the control of the underlying cause. Mild examples may cause few problems. If the swelling becomes a cosmetic concern, partial parotidectomy can be performed. Pilocarpine recently has been reported to be beneficial in the treatment of bulimic patients with sialadenosis.

Systemic conditions with salivary gland involvement

Many systemic diseases are manifested by salivary gland dysfunction. The most prominent example is Sjögren's syndrome. Xerostomia, the symptom of oral dryness, has been reported in association with many additional systemic conditions. In some instances, it is unclear whether these symptoms and the salivary gland changes are part of the disease process or whether they result from treatment of the disease.

Metabolic Conditions

The underlying systemic metabolic disorders that are commonly associated with salivary gland disease include diabetes, anorexia nervosa, bulimia, and alcoholism. The parotid gland is not often involved.

DIABETES

Diabetes mellitus is a common endocrine disease, especially in the geriatric population. Multiple metabolic abnormalities take place, and long-term complications such as renal hypertension, neuropathies, and ophthalmic disease can occur. Patients with uncontrolled diabetes often report dry mouth, which is believed to be due to Polyuria and poor hydration. Research results regarding salivary flow and compositional changes in diabetic patients are contradictory. One study reported that salivary flow rates in children with poorly controlled diabetes mellitus were decreased when compared to flow rates in well-controlled pediatric diabetic patients and normal controls. However, other investigators found that salivary flow rates were normal but that salivary compositional changes occurred in pediatric diabetic patients. Ship and colleagues conducted a clinical trial comparing adult diabetes type 2 patients with normal controls. They found that patients with poorly controlled diabetes had lower salivary flow rates when compared to patients with well-controlled diabetes and to normal controls. Of interest, these investigators also found that there was no difference between these populations in the frequency of xerostomic complaints, and further, that salivary dysfunction may be present in older diabetic patients who do not complaint of xerostomia. The etiology of diabetic salivary gland dysfunction is unclear. Sreebny and colleagues suggested that poor glycemic control directly effects salivary gland metabolism. It has also been suggested that autonomic nervous system dysfunction may play a role. Meurman and colleagues reported no change in flow rates between non-insulin dependent diabetic patients and normal controls. However, they found the effects of xerostomic medications on salivary flow rates to be stronger in the diabetic patients. They postulated that this was due to documented autonomic nervous system dysfunction in the diabetic population.

ANOREXIA NERVOSA

Salivary gland enlargement and dysfunction can occur in patients with anorexia nervosa and bulimia. The enlargement appears to be related to nutritional deficiencies and to the habit of induced vomiting. One case study reported that histologic examination of the involved salivary gland revealed acinar enlargement and reduced interstitial fat. Salivary gland enlargement usually resolves when patients return to normal weight and discontinue unhealthy eating habits. However, benign hypertrophy may persist and be a cosmetic concern. While superficial parotidectomy will reduce salivary hypertrophy, some surgeons believe that surgical management is contraindicated for a patient with an eating disorder, because of the increased risk associated with the patient's metabolic imbalance and psychological profile.

Total and salivary specific amylase levels are increased with bulimia. Salivary amylase tends to increase with the frequency of binge eating, but the correlation is not strong enough to include salivary amylase levels as an index of disease severity. Eating disorders are difficult to diagnose because of the secretive nature of the condition. To facilitate early diagnosis and treatment, dentists should be aware of the common oral findings (enamel erosion, xerostomia, salivary gland enlargement, mucosal erythema, and cheilitis). Patients should be questioned directly if an eating disorder is suspected. Eating disorders must be considered in the differential diagnosis of salivary gland dysfunction and hypertrophy.

CHRONIC ALCOHOLISM

Chronic alcoholism is associated with salivary gland dysfunction and bilateral salivary (usually parotid) gland enlargement. The exact etiology is unclear, but the decreased salivary flow is believed to be due to dehydration and poor nutrition. Enlarged salivary glands in alcoholic patients demonstrate fatty-tissue changes on histologic examination.

Medication-induced salivary dysfunction

There are over 400 medications that are listed as having dry mouth as an adverse event. However, there are relatively few drugs that have been shown objectively to reduce salivary function. The reason for this disparity is unclear. It may be due to unrecognized alterations in saliva composition that lead to the perception of oral dryness in spite of an apparently unchanged volume of saliva .Drugs that have been shown to result in salivary dysfunction include anticholinergics, antidepressants (particularly tricyclics), antihypertensives, and antihistaminics. Medication-induced salivary hypo function usually affects the unstimulated output, leaving stimulated function intact. When the causative drug is withdrawn, function often returns to normal.

Granulomatous Conditions

Tuberculosis

Tuberculosis (TB) is a chronic bacterial infection, caused by Mycobacterium tuberculosis that leads to the formation of granulomas in the infected tissues. The lungs are most commonly affected, but other tissues, including the salivary glands, may be involved. Patients with TB may experience xerostomia and/or salivary gland swelling, with granuloma or cyst formation within the affected glands. Salivary gland enlargement usually presents as part of a characteristic symptom complex; however, salivary gland changes have been reported in the absence of systemic symptoms. The worldwide increase in mycobacterial diseases and their association with immunocompromised patients must be considered when developing a differential diagnosis. Diagnosis depends on the identification of Mycobacterium. Treatment of the salivary involvement is encompassed in standard multidrug anti-TB chemotherapy. Patients who have not responded to appropriate chemotherapy regimens have required surgical intervention to address persistent salivary gland pathology.

Sarcoidosis

Etiology

Sarcoidosis is a granulomatous disease of undetermined origin. Although no specific cause has been identified, it has been suggested that this disease represents an infection or a hypersensitivity response to atypical mycobacteria. As many as 90% of patients in some studies showed significant titers of serum antibodies to these organisms. In some patients with sarcoidosis, a transmissible agent from human sarcoid tissue has been identified. With the use of molecular biologic techniques, mycobacterial DNA and RNA have been identified in sarcoid tissues, raising the possibility of Mycobacterium tuberculosis or a related organism as a causative agent. Susceptibility related to human leukocyte antigens (HLAs) has been studied. Patients with some histocompatibility antigens (HLA-B7, HLA-B5, and HLA-A9) may have a greater incidence of sarcoidosis than do others. It has also been found that most patients with sarcoidosis are anergic, demonstrating decreased levels of cutaneous sensitization to dinitrochlorobenzene, as well as to tuberculin, mumps virus, Candida antigen, and pertussis antigen. Sarcoidosis is a chronic condition in which T lymphocytes, mononuclear phagocytes, and granulomas cause destruction of involved tissue.

Clinical Features

The manifestations of this disease are well known. Clinical courses range from spontaneous resolution to chronic progression. The disease may affect individuals at any age, although most are affected in the second through fourth decades. Females show a higher incidence than do males, and African-Americans are more commonly affected than whites. Sarcoidosis is usually a self-limiting, benign disease with an insidious onset and protracted course. Patients may complain of lethargy, chronic fatigue, and anorexia, with specific signs and symptoms related to the organ involved. Pulmonary manifestations are the most characteristic of this disease. They are typified by bilateral, hilar, and less commonly, paratracheal lymphadenopathy. The disease may stabilize at this point, or it may advance to pulmonary fibrosis and a more ominous prognosis. The most serious complications of sarcoidosis are pulmonary hypertension, respiratory failure and corpulmonale.

The skin may be involved in approximately 25% of cases; most commonly, an erythema nodosum of acute onset and short duration is seen. Skin plaques characterized by nontender, dark purple, elevated areas on the limbs, abdomen, and buttocks may appear. Another form of cutaneous pathology includes lesions known as lupus pernio, a term used to describe symmetric, infiltrative, violaceous plaques on the nose, cheeks, ears, forehead, and hands. Ocular involvement is variable, with inflammation of the anterior uveal tract most commonly seen. This may be associated with parotid gland swelling and fever, so-called uveoparotid fever or Heerfordt's syndrome.

Hepatic involvement is quite common, with approximately 60% of patients showing granulomatous lesions on liver biopsy specimens. However, clinical evidence of hepatic involvement appears in fewer than 50% of patients, as demonstrated in abnormal liver function test results. Osseous lesions are uncommonly noted, with a 5% occurrence rate in most studies. When present, punched-out lesions involving the distal phalanges with erosions of cancellous bone and an intact cortex are seen. Destruction of alveolar bone with tooth mobility may be evident within the maxilla and mandible. Oral soft tissue lesions of sarcoidosis are nodular and generally indistinguishable from those seen in Crohn's disease. Parotid swelling may occur either unilaterally or bilaterally with about equal frequency. This is often associated with lassitude, fever, gastrointestinal upset, joint pains, and night sweats, which may precede glandular involvement by several days to weeks. Other salivary glands may also be involved in the granulomatous inflammatory process, leading to xerostomia. The upper aerodigestive tract maybe involved, with lesions developing in the nasal mucosa, especially in the inferior turbinate and septal regions. Granulomas may also occur in the nasal sinuses, pharynx, epiglottis, and larynx. Serum chemistry, radiographic studies, and biopsy are useful laboratory tests. Serum chemistry studies should include calcium (for evidence of hypercalcemia) and angiotensin I-converting enzyme, lysozyme, and adenosine deaminase levels (for evidence of macrophage activity within granulomas. Gallium scintiscanning and routine chest radiographs and intraoral films may be used to demonstrate bone involvement.

Histopathology

Consistent microscopic findings of sarcoidosis are noncaseating granulomas. The granulomas may be well demarcated and discrete or confluent. Within the granulomas are epithelioid macrophages and multinucleated giant cells, which may contain stellate inclusions (asteroid bodies) and concentrically laminar calcifications (Schaumann bodies). A diffuse lymphocytic infiltrate may be seen around the periphery of the granulomas. Absent is the caseation-type necrosis that is typical of tuberculosis. Microorganisms are also absent. A lip biopsy may occasionally provide evidence of sarcoid involvement of minor salivary glands in support of a clinical impression of pulmonary disease.

Diagnosis

The Kveim test has traditionally been used to establish the diagnosis of sarcoidosis; however, this test is no longer used. Of considerable value is a laboratory assay for Angiotensin I-Converting Enzyme. Elevation of this enzyme in conjunction with a positive chest radiograph has a high diagnostic reliability. The histologic differential diagnosis includes tuberculosis, Crohn's disease, leprosy, cat-scratch disease, fungal infections (blastomycosis, coccidioidomycosis and histoplasmosis), and parasitic diseases such as toxoplasmosis. Granulomas seen in association with beryllium and talc exposure must also be considered.

Treatment and Prognosis

Spontaneous resolution occurs in a significant number of patients. Corticosteroids are generally considered beneficial and remain the drugs of choice in treating symptomatic pulmonary sarcoidosis. Other agents may be used in addition to or instead of corticosteroids. Chloroquine has been found to be useful in the management of this disease, either alone or in combination with corticosteroids. Immunosuppressive drugs have been used with good results in individuals not responding to corticosteroid management. Immimomodulators such as levamisole may be useful in the management of arthritic symptoms caused by sarcoidosis.

In general, the prognosis for sarcoidosis is good, but patients must be monitored periodically with chest radiographs and serum Angiotensin I-Converting Enzyme determinations. Clinical relapses are not usual in cases in which spontaneous resolution has occurred.

Immune Conditions

BENIGN LYMPHOEPITHELIAL LESION (MIKULICZ'S DISEASE)

In the late 1800s, Johann von Mikulicz-Radecki described the case of a patient with an unusual bilateral painless swelling of the lacrimal glands and all of the salivary glands. Histopathologic examination of the involved glands showed an intense lymphocytic infiltrate, with features that today arc recognized microscopically as the benign lymphoepithelial lesion. This clinical presentation became known as Mikulicz disease, and clinicians began using this term to describe a variety of cases of bilateral parotid and lacrimal enlargement. However, many of these cases were not examples of benign lymphoepithelial lesions microscopically; instead, they represented salivary and lacrimal involvement by other disease processes, such as tuberculosis, sarcoidosis, and lymphoma. These cases of parotid and lacrimal enlargement secondary to other diseases were later recognized as being different and termed Mikulicz syndrome, with the term Mikulicz disease reserved for cases associated with benign lymphoepithelial lesions. However, these two terms have become so confusing and ambiguous that they should no longer be used. Many cases of so-called Mikulicz disease may be examples of what is now more commonly known as Sjogren syndrome. Sjogren syndrome is an autoimmune disease that may produce bilateral salivary and lacrimal enlargement, with microscopic features of benign lymphoepithelial lesion. However, not all benign lymphoepithelial lesions are necessarily associated with the clinical disease complex of Sjogren syndrome.

Clinical Features

The etiology of benign lymphoepithelial lesion is unknown. It has been speculated that autoimmune, viral, or genetic factors are the trigger. Patients present with unilateral or bilateral salivary gland swelling due to a benign lymphoid infiltration. Reduced salivary flow makes these patients susceptible to salivary gland infections. Most benign lymphoepithelial lesions develop as a component of Sjogren syndrome. Those not associated with Sjogren syndrome are usually unilateral, although occasional bilateral examples are seen. On occasion, benign lymphoepithelial lesions occur in association with other salivary gland pathologic conditions, such as sialoliths and benign or malignant epithelial tumors.

The benign lymphoepithelial lesion most often develops in adults, with a mean age of 50 years. From 60% to 80% of cases occur in women. Eighty-five percent of cases occur in the parotid gland, with infrequent examples also reported in the submandibular gland and minor salivary glands. The lesion usually appears as a firm, diffuse swelling of the affected gland that sometimes is dramatic in size. It may be asymptomatic or associated with mild pain.

Histopathologic Features

Microscopic examination of the benign lymphoepithelial lesion shows a heavy lymphocytic infiltrate associated with the destruction of the salivary acini. Germinal centers may or may not be seen. Although the acini are destroyed, the ductal epithelium persists. The ductal cells and surrounding myoepithelial cells become hyperplastic, forming highly characteristic groups of cells, known as epimyoepithelial islands, throughout the lymphoid proliferation. The presence of epimyoepithelial islands once was considered indicative of a benign process, but now it is recognized that these islands also can be found in low-grade salivary lymphomas of the mucosa-associated lymphoid tissue (MALT lymphomas)

Treatment and Prognosis

The differential diagnosis includes Sjögren's syndrome, lymphoma, sarcoidosis, and other diseases associated with salivary gland enlargement. Diagnosis is based on findings of salivary gland biopsy and the absence of the abnormalities in peripheral blood counts and autoimmune serologies seen in Sjögren's syndrome. Although the benign lymphoepithelial lesion frequently necessitates surgical removal of the involved gland, the prognosis in most cases is good. However, individuals with benign lymphoepithelial lesion have an increased risk for lymphoma, either within the affected gland or in an extra salivary site. Although the exact risk is uncertain, one study showed the risk in patients with Sjogren syndrome to be more than 40 times higher than expected in the general population. With the development of modern molecular techniques to assess for gene rearrangements and mono-clonality within lymphoid infiltrates, it is now recognized that some lesions originally believed to represent benign lymphoepithelial lesions are actually early-stage MALT lymphomas. Many experts now recognize a spectrum of salivary lymphoid proliferations, which range from benign lymphoepithelial lesions to borderline lesions to frank lymphomas. Because of this, some authors have dropped the term "benign" from this spectrum and refer to these proliferations only as lymphoepithelial lesions. Fortunately, most MALT lymphomas are low-grade tumors that tend to remain localized with good survival rates. However, occasional tumors transform to higher-grade lymphomas with more aggressive behavior.

In addition, a rare malignant counterpart of this lesion, called a malignant lymphoepithelial lesion or lymphoepithelial carcinoma, represents a poorly differentiated salivary carcinoma with a prominent lymphoid stroma. Most of these lesions have occurred in Inuits (Eskimos) and Asians and appear to have arisen de novo as carcinomas; however, some cases (especially in non-Inuits) have been reported to develop from a prior benign lymphoepithelial lesion. Because of the strong ethnic association of this tumor, attempts have been made to determine a common causative agent. Most of this speculation has centered on the Epstein-Barr virus, although definite proof has not been established. The prognosis for these carcinomas appears guarded, although Asian patients have had a better survival rate.

SJOGREN SYNDROME

Sjogren syndrome is a chronic, systemic autoimmune disorder that principally involves the salivary and lacrimal glands, resulting in xerostomia (dry mouth) and xerophthalmia (dry eyes). The effects on the eye often are called keratoconjunctivitis Sicca (Sicca = dry), and the clinical presentation of both xerostomia and xerophthalmia is also sometimes called the sicca syndrome. Two forms of the disease are recognized:

1. Primary Sjogren syndrome (sicca syndrome alone; no other autoimmune disorder is present)
2. Secondary Sjogren syndrome (the patient manifests sicca syndrome in addition to another associated autoimmune disease)

The cause of Sjogren syndrome is unknown. Although it is not a hereditary disease per se, there is evidence of a genetic influence. Relatives of affected patients have an increased frequency of other autoimmune diseases. In addition, certain histocompatibility antigens (HLAs) are found with greater frequency in patients with Sjogren syndrome. HLA-DRw52 is associated with both forms of the disease; HLA-B8 and HLA-DR3 are seen with increased frequency in the primary form of the disease. It has been suggested that viruses, such as Epstein-Barr virus or human T cell lymphotropic virus, may play a pathogenetic role in Sjogren syndrome, but evidence for this is still speculative.

Clinical and Radiographic Features

Sjogren syndrome is not a rare condition. Although the exact prevalence is unknown, estimates have ranged from 0.2% to 3.0%, depending on the population studied and the clinical criteria used. Application of the stricter San Diego criteria results in a lower prevalence rate than the European Economic Community criteria. Between 80% and 90% of cases of Sjogren syndrome occur in females. It is seen predominantly in middle-aged adults, but rare examples have been described in children.

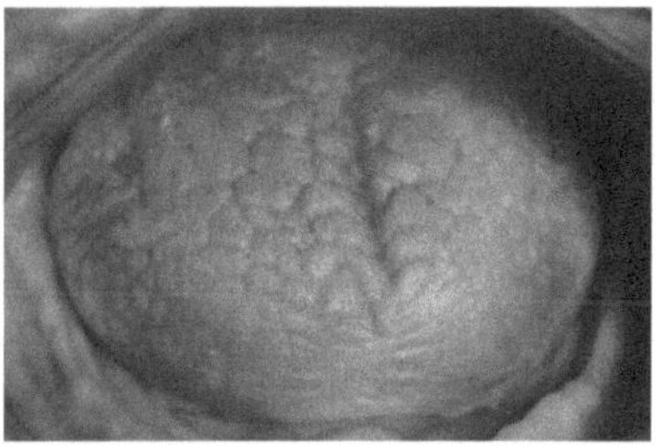

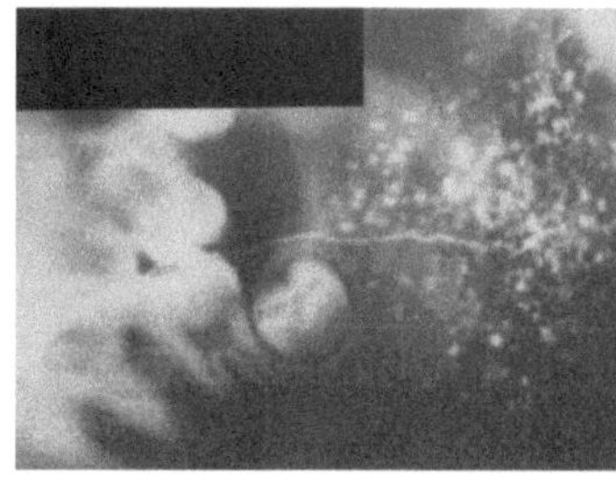

San Diego Criteria for Sjogren Syndrome

I. Primary Sjogren syndrome

A. Symptoms and objective signs of ocular dryness

1. Schirmer's test less than 8 mm wetting per 5 minutes, AND
2. Positive Rose Bengal staining of cornea or conjunctiva to demonstrate keratoconjunctivitis sicca.

B. Symptoms and objective signs of dry mouth

1. Decreased parotid flow rate using Lashley cups or other methods, AND
2. Abnormal findings from biopsy of minor salivary gland (focus score of S2 based on average of four evaluable lobules).

C. Serologic evidence of a systemic autoimmunity

1. Elevated rheumatoid factor > 1:320, OR
2. Elevated antinuclear antibody (ANA) > 1:320, OR
3. Presence of anti-SS-A (Ro) or anti-SS-B (La) antibodies

II. Secondary Sjogren syndrome

Characteristic signs and symptoms of Sjogren syndrome (as previously described), plus clinical features sufficient to allow a diagnosis of rheumatoid arthritis, systemic lupus erythematosus, polymyositis, scleroderma, or biliary cirrhosis. Exclusions: sarcoidosis, preexisting lymphoma, human immunodeficiency virus (HIV), hepatitis B or C, primary fibromyalgia, and other known causes of autonomic neuropathy, keratitis sicca, or salivary gland enlargement.

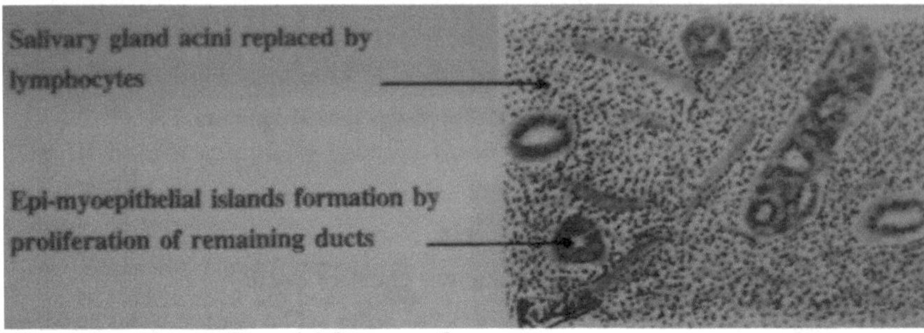

Sjogren's syndrome: Potential Organopathy

SKIN

Dryness (reduced sweat production)

Scleroderma

Lupus erythematosus

SALIVARY AND LACRIMAL GLANDS

Enlargement

Xerostomia, dental caries, candidiasis

Keratoconjunctivitis sicca

GASTROINTESTINAL TRACT

Biliary cirrhosis Hepatitis

RESPIRATORY TRACT

Rhinitis, pharyngitis Obstructive pulmonary disease

CARDIOVASCULAR SYSTEM

Vasculitis

MUSCULOSKELETAL SYSTEM

Rheumatoid arthritis Myositis

HEMATOPOIETIC SYSTEM

Lymphoma Anemia, leucopenia

When the condition is associated with another connective tissue disease, it is called secondary Sjogren syndrome. It can be associated with almost any other autoimmune disease, but the most common associated disorder is rheumatoid arthritis. About 15% of patients with rheumatoid arthritis have Sjogren syndrome. In addition, secondary Sjogren syndrome may develop in 30% of patients with systemic lupus erythematosus.

The principal oral symptom is xerostomia, which is caused by decreased salivary secretions; however, the severity of this dryness can vary widely from patient to patient. The saliva may appear frothy, with a lack of the usual pooling saliva in the floor of the mouth. Affected patients may complain of difficulty in swallowing, altered taste, or difficulty in wearing dentures. The tongue often becomes fissured and exhibits atrophy of the papillae. The oral mucosa may be red and tender, usually as a result of secondary candidiasis. Related denture sore mouth and angular cheilitis are common. The lack of salivary cleansing action predisposes the patient to dental decay, especially cervical caries.

From one third to one half of patients have diffuse, firm enlargement of the major salivary glands during the course of their disease. This swelling is usually bilateral, may be nonpainful or slightly tender, and may be intermittent or persistent in nature. The greater the severity of the disease, the greater the likelihood of this salivary enlargement. In addition, the reduced salivary flow places these individuals at increased risk for retrograde bacterial sialadenitis.

Although it is not diagnostic, sialographic examination often reveals punctate sialectasia and lack of normal arborization of the ductal system, typically demonstrating a "fruit-laden, branchless tree" pattern. Scintigraphy with radioactive technetium-99 in pertechnetate characteristically shows decreased uptake and delayed emptying of the isotope.

The term keratoconjunctivitis sicca describes not only the reduced tear production by the lacrimal glands but also the pathologic effect on the epithelial cells of the ocular surface. As in xerostomia, the severity of xerophthalmia can vary widely from one patient to the next. The lacrimal inflammation causes a decreased the aqueous layer of the tear film; however, mucin production is normal and may result in a mucoid discharge Patients often complain of a scratchy, gritty sensation or the perceived presence of a foreign body in them. Defects of the ocular surface epithelium develop and can be demonstrated with rose bengal dye. Vision nay become blurred, and sometimes there is an aching pain. The ocular manifestations are least severe in the morning on wakening and become more pronounced as the day progresses.

A simple means to confirm the decreased tear secretion is the Schirmer test. Standardized strips of sterile filter paper arc placed over the margins of the lower lids so that their tabbed ends rest just inside the lower lid, By measuring the length of wetting of the filter paper, tear production can be assessed. Values below 5 mm (after a 5-minute period) are highly suggestive of keratoconjunctivitis sicca, and values from 0 to 2 mm strongly confirm a dry-eye state.

Sjogren syndrome is a systemic disease, and the inflammatory process also can affect various other body tissues. The skin is often dry, as are the nasal and vaginal mucosae. Fatigue is fairly common, and depression sometimes can occur. Other possible associated problems include lymphadenopathy, primary biliary cirrhosis, Raynaud's phenomenon, interstitial nephritis, interstitial lungfibrosis, vasculitis, and peripheral neuropathies.

Laboratory Values

In patients with Sjogren syndrome, the erythrocyte sedimentation rate is high and serum immunoglobulin levels, especially IgG, typically are elevated. A variety of autoantibodies can be produced, and although none of these is specifically diagnostic, their presence can be another helpful clue to the diagnosis. A positive rheumatoid factor (RF) is found in 75% of cases, regardless of whether the patient has rheumatoid arthritis. Antinuclear antibodies (ANA) are also present in most patients. Two particular nuclear autoantibodies—anti-SS-A (anti-Roland anti-SS-6 (anti-La)—frequently are found, especially in patients with primary Sjogren syndrome. Occasionally, salivary duct autoantibodies also can be demonstrated, usually in secondary Sjogren syndrome. However, because these are infrequent in primary cases, they are believed to occur as a secondary phenomenon (rather than playing a primary role in pathogenesis). Several studies have suggested that salivary protein electrophoresis is a potentially useful test for the diagnosis of Sjogren syndrome.

Histopathologic Features

The basic microscopic finding in Sjogren syndrome is a lymphocytic infiltration of the salivary glands, with destruction of the acinar units. If the major glands are enlarged, microscopic examination usually shows progression to a lymphoepithelial lesion, with characteristic epimyoepithelial islands in a background lymphoid stroma. Lymphocytic infiltration of the minor glands also occurs, although epimyoepithelial islands are rarely seen in this location.

Biopsy of the minor salivary glands of the lower lip has become a useful test in the diagnosis of Sjogren syndrome. A 1.5 to 2.0 cm incision is made on clinically normal lower labial mucosa, parallel to the vermilion border and lateral to the midline, allowing the harvest of five or more accessory glands. These glands then are examined histopathologically for the presence of focal chronic inflammatory aggregates (50 or more lymphocytes and plasma cells). These aggregates should be adjacent to normal-appearing acini and should be found consistently in most of the glands in the specimen. The finding of more than one focus of 50 or more cells within a 4mm area of glandular tissue is considered supportive of the diagnosis of Sjogren syndrome. The greater the number of foci (upto10 or confluent foci), the greater the correlation with this diagnosis. The focal nature of this chronic inflammation among otherwise normal acini is a highly suggestive pattern; in contrast, the finding of scattered inflammation with ductal dilatation and fibrosis (chronic sclerosing sialadenitis) does not support the diagnosis of Sjogren syndrome. Although labial salivary gland biopsy has become a widely used test in the diagnosis of Sjogren syndrome, it is not 100% reliable. Some patients diagnosed with Sjogren syndrome will show no significant labial gland inflammation; conversely, examination of labial glands removed incidentally from non-Sjogren patients sometimes will show focal lymphocytic infiltrates. Other authors have advocated incisional biopsy of the parotid gland through a posterior auricular approach instead of a labial salivary gland biopsy. One study has shown this technique to be more sensitive in demonstrating inflammatory changes that support the diagnosis of Sjogren syndrome; however, other authors think that this technique confers no increased benefit over labial gland biopsy. Parotid biopsy may enable the clinician to evaluate an enlarged gland for the development of lymphoma and rule out the possibility of sialadenosis or sarcoidosis.

Diagnosis

There are no universally accepted diagnostic criteria for SS, and multiple criteria sets have been published. The strictest criteria include objective measurement of decreased salivary and lacrimal gland function, positive autoimmune serologies, and a minor salivary gland biopsy specimen that demonstrates focal mononuclear cell infiltration in a periductal pattern (focus score > 1. Less stringent criteria, which rely partly on symptomatic reports, exist and are commonly used by clinicians. At present, a criteria set created by a European Community SS multicenter study group and validated by large-scale clinical testing is gaining wider acceptance. Efforts are being made to establish an internationally accepted diagnostic criteria set for SS. Most investigators accept the premise that a definitive diagnosis of primary SS requires either the presence of a salivary gland biopsy specimen demonstrating characteristic histopathologic findings or the presence of autoantibodies against the extractable nuclear antigens SS-A/Ro or SS-B/La, in addition to objective evidence of lacrimal dysfunction. The minor salivary gland biopsy specimen finding is considered to be the best sole diagnostic criterion for the salivary component of SS. A grading system exists for quantifying the salivary histologic changes seen in the minor glands in SS, as follows: (1) The numbers of infiltrating mononuclear cells are determined, with an aggregate of 50 or more cells being termed a focus;

(2) The total number of foci and the surface area of the specimen are measured; and

(3) The number of foci per 4 mm2 is calculated.

This constitutes the focus score. The range is from 0 to 12, with 12 denoting confluent infiltrates. A focus score of 1 is considered positive for SS in some criteria although others require the score to be > 1. Acinar degeneration, with the relative preservation of ductal structures, is also noted. Sialography shows characteristic changes and may be useful in the evaluation of SS. MRI or CT can be helpful also, particularly in the assessment of enlarged glands and potential lymphadenopathies. MRI is preferable to CT, unless a stone or other calcified structure requires visualization as MRI provides better resolution of soft tissue. Some clinicians use Tc-99m radionuclide studies to determine salivary gland function.

Treatment and Prognosis

The treatment of the patient with Sjogren syndrome is mostly supportive. The dry eyes are best managed by periodic use of artificial tears; in addition, attempts can be made to conserve the tear film through the use of sealed glasses to prevent evaporation. Sealing the lacrimal punctum at the inner margin of the eyelids also can be helpful by blocking of the normal drainage of any lacrimal secretions into the nose.

Artificial saliva is available for the treatment of xerostomia; sugarless candy or gum can help to keep the mouth moist. Symptoms often can be relieved by the use of oral hygiene products that contain lactoperoxidase, lysozyme, and lactoferrin (e.g., Biotene toothpaste and mouth rinse; Oralbalance gel). Sialagogues, such as pilocarpine and cevimeline can be useful to stimulate salivary flow if enough functional salivary tissue still remains. Medications known to diminish secretions should be avoided, if at all possible. Because of the increased risk of dental caries, daily fluoride applications may be indicated in dentulous patients. Antifungal therapy often is needed to treat secondary candidiasis.

Patients with Sjogren syndrome have an increased risk for lymphoma, up to 40 times higher than the normal population. These tumors may arise initially within the salivary glands or within lymph nodes. With the advent of modern molecular pathology techniques to detect B-cell monoclonality (e.g., in situ hybridization, polymerase chain reaction [PCR]), many salivary gland infiltrates formerly thought to represent benign lymphoepithelial lesions are now being diagnosed as lymphomas. These tumors are predominantly low-grade non-Hodgkin's B-cell lymphomas of the mucosa-associated lymphoid tissue (MALT lymphomas), although occasionally, high-grade MALT lymphomas can develop which demonstrate more aggressive behavior. The detection of immunoglobulin gene rearrangements in labial salivary gland biopsies may prove to be a useful marker for predicting the development of lymphoma.

Sialolithiasis (Salivary Stones)

The true prevalence of sialolithiasis is difficult to determine since many cases are asymptomatic. Sialoliths are calcified and organic matter that forms within the secretory system of the major salivary glands. The etiology of sialolith formation is still unknown; however, there are several factors that contribute to stone formation. Inflammation, irregularities in the duct system, local irritants, and anticholinergic medications may cause pooling of saliva within the duct, which is thought to promote stone formation. . It is believed that a nidus of salivary organic material becomes calcified and gradually forms a sialolith .Researchers have investigated the possibility of altered salivary hydrogen ion concentration (pH), abnormal serum calcium and phosphorous levels, and diet as causes of sialolith formation, but consistent alterations have not been detected. Frequently, there is no clear explanation for stone formation. Since the underlying cause is unknown and uncorrected in most patients, the recurrence rate is ≈20%. It is known that the structure of sialoliths is crystalline and that sialoliths are primarily composed of hydroxyapatite. The chemical composition is calcium phosphate and carbon, with trace amounts of magnesium, potassium chloride, and ammonium. Fifty percent of parotid gland sialoliths and 20% of submandibular gland sialoliths are poorly calcified. This is clinically significant because such sialoliths are not radiographically detectable. The submandibular gland is the most common site of involvement, and 80 to 90% of sialoliths occur in this gland. The parotid gland is involved in 5 to 15% of cases, and 2 to 5% of cases occur in the sublingual or minor salivary glands. It is believed that the higher rate of sialolith formation in the submandibular gland is due to

(1) The torturous course of Wharton's duct,

(2) Higher calcium and phosphate levels, and

(3) The dependent position of the submandibular glands, which leave them prone to stasis.

Gout can cause salivary calculi composed of uric acid. However, patients with a history of renal stone formation do not have an increased incidence of salivary gland stone formation. There is one report of obstructive sialadenitis by intraparotid deposits of gold salts in a patient receiving sodium aurothiomalate (gold salt compound) treatment for rheumatoid arthritis.

Clinical presentation and Evaluation

Patients with sialoliths most commonly present with a history of acute, painful, and intermittent swelling of the affected major salivary gland. The degree of symptoms is dependent on the extent of salivary duct obstruction and the presence of secondary infection. Typically, eating will initiate the salivary gland swelling. The stone totally or partially blocks the flow of saliva, causing salivary pooling within the ducts and gland body. Since the glands are encapsulated, there is little space for expansion, and enlargement causes pain. If the calculus partially blocks the duct, then the swelling subsides as salivary stimulation is removed and output decreases, and saliva seeps past the partial obstruction. The involved gland is usually enlarged and tender. Stasis of the saliva may lead to infection, fibrosis, and gland atrophy. Fistulae, a sinus tract, or ulceration may occur over the stone in chronic cases. An examination of the soft tissue surrounding the duct may show a severe inflammatory reaction.

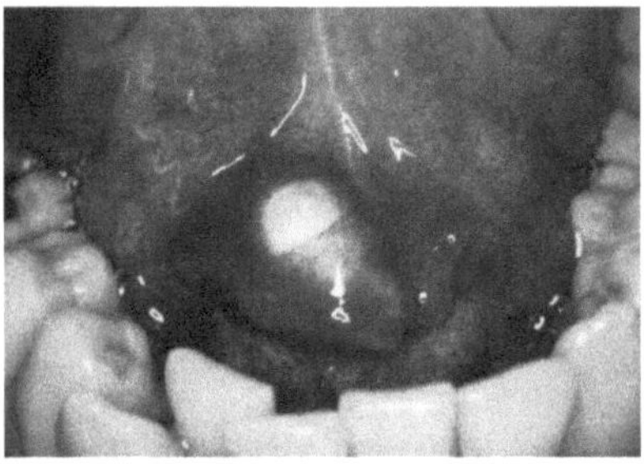

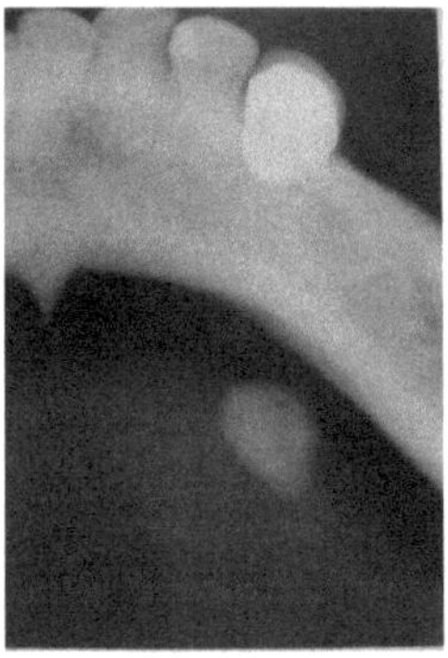

Palpation along the pathway of the duct may confirm the presence of a stone. Bacterial infections may or may not be superimposed and are more common with chronic obstructions. Other complications from sialoliths include acute sialadenitis, ductal stricter and ductal dilatation. Radiographic examination is often necessary since the stone may not be accessible to bimanual palpation. However, as stated earlier, poorly calcified sialoliths will not be visible radiographically. An occlusal view is the recommended view for radiography of submandibular glands. Stones in the parotid gland can be more difficult to visualize due to the superimposition of other anatomic structures; therefore, requesting proper radiographic views is important. An anteroposterior view of the face is useful for visualization of a parotid stone. One can also place an occlusal film intraorally adjacent to the duct. CT may be used for the detection of sialoliths and has 10 times the sensitivity of plain-film radiography for detecting calcifications. Sialoliths typically appear as radiopaque masses on radiographic examination. However, not all stones are visible on standard radiographs (perhaps because of the degree of calcification of some lesions). They may be discovered anywhere along the length of the duct or within the gland itself. Stones in the terminal portion of the sub-mandibular duct are best demonstrated with an occlusal radiograph. On panoramic or periapical radiographs, the calcification may appear superimposed on the mandible and care must be exercised not to confuse it with an intrabony lesion. Multiple parotid stones radiographically can mimic calcified parotid lymph nodes, such as might occur in tuberculosis. Sialography, ultrasound, and computed tomography (CT) scanning may be helpful additional imaging studies for sialoliths.

Calcified phleboliths are stones that lie within a blood vessel; they can be easily mistaken radiographically for sialoliths. Phleboliths occur outside the ductal structure, and sialography can therefore aid in differentiating these lesions. Stanley and colleagues reported using FNA of the submandibular gland as a diagnostic tool in 5 patients who did not present with classic symptoms of sialolithiasis. In 3 of the 5 cases, stone fragments were identified, and the patients were diagnosed with sialolithiasis. In the other 2 patients, FNA samples did not reveal stone fragments but showed foam cells and metaplastic squamous cells in a mucoid background that resembled low-grade mucoepidermoid carcinoma. Surgical excision of the glands was performed, and stones were found, which emphasizes that FNA cytology should be interpreted cautiously in this situation.

Sialoliths also can form within the minor salivary glands, most often within the glands of the upper lip or buccal mucosa .Salivary stones can occur at almost any age, but they are most common in young and middle-aged adults. Minor gland sialoliths often are asymptomatic but may produce local swelling or tenderness of the affected gland. A small radiopacity often can be demonstrated with a soft tissue radiograph.

Histopathologic Features

On gross examination, sialoliths appear as hard masses that are round, oval, or cylindrical. They are typically yellow, although they may be white or yellowish-brown. Submandibular stones tend to be larger than those of the parotid or minor glands. Sialoliths are usually solitary, although occasionally two or more stones may be discovered at surgery.

TREATMENT

During the acute phase, therapy is primarily supportive. Standard care includes analgesics, hydration, antibiotics, and antipyretics, as necessary. In pronounced exacerbations, surgical intervention for drainage is sometimes required. Stones at or near the orifice of the duct can often be removed transorally by milking the gland, but deeper stones require surgery. Once the acute phase subsides, surgical treatment can be performed. Location within the duct determines the type of surgery required for removal of the stone. If the stone lies in the intraglandular portion of the duct, it is recommended that the entire gland be removed. As much as 75% of normal function can return if the stone can be removed from within the duct, without entering the body of the gland. Lithotripsy is gaining popularity because it offers a noninvasive treatment for sialoliths. Current protocols use ultrasonography to detect the stone and extracorporeal lithotripsy to fragment the stone. Several treatments may be needed, and a stone with a diameter of > 2 mm is required for detection with ultrasonography. Reported complications associated with this procedure include transient hearing changes, hematoma at the site, and pain. There have been initial reports of intraductal lithotripsy, but this technique requires specialized equipment and has been performed at only a few centers.

.

Mucoceles

"Mucocele"is a clinical term that describes swelling caused by the accumulation of saliva at the site of a traumatized or obstructed minor salivary gland duct. Mucoceles are classified as extravasation types and retention types. . Because each has a distinctive pathogenesis and microscopy, they are considered separately. A large form of mucocele located in the floor of the mouth is known as a ranula.

The mucocele is a common lesion of the oral mucosa that results from rupture of a salivary gland duct and mucin into the surrounding soft tissues. This spillage is often the result of local trauma, although there is no known history of trauma in many cases. Unlike the salivary duct cyst, the mucocele is not a true cyst because it lacks an epithelial lining. Some authors, however, have included true salivary duct cysts in their reported series of "mucoceles." Because these two entities exhibit distinctly different clinical and histopathologic features, they are discussed as separate.

Clinical Features

Mucoceles typically appear as dome-shaped mucosal swellings that can range from 1 or 2 mm to several centimeters in size .They are most common in children and young adults, perhaps because younger people are more likely to experience trauma that induces mucin spillage. However, mucoceles have been reported in patients of all ages, including newborn infants and older people. The spilled mucin below the mucosal surface often imparts a bluish translucent hue to the swelling, although deeper mucoceles may be normal in color. The lesion characteristically is fluctuant, but some mucoceles feel firmer to palpation. The reported duration of the lesion can vary from a few days to several years; most patients report that the lesion has been present for several weeks. Many patients relate a history of a recurrent swelling that periodically may rupture and release its fluid contents.

The lower lip is the most common site for e mucocele, accounting for over 60% of all cases. Mucoceles usually are found lateral to the midline. Less common sites include the buccal mucosa, anterior ventral tongue, and floor of mouth (ranula). Mucoceles rarely develop on the upper lip. This is in contradistinction to salivary gland tumors, which are not unusual in the upper lip but are distinctly uncommon in the lower lip. The soft palate and retromolar area are also uncommon sites for mucoceles. However, one interesting variant, the superficial mucocele, does develop in these areas and along the posterior buccal mucosa. Superficial mucoceles present as single or multiple tense vesicles that measure 1 to 4 mm in diameter. The lesions often burst, leaving shallow, painful ulcers that heal within a few days.

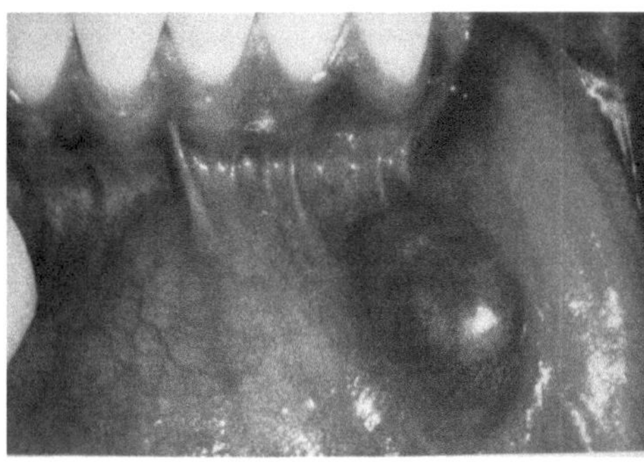

Repeated episodes at the same location are not unusual. Some patients relate the development of the lesions to mealtimes. The vesicular appearance is created by the superficial nature of the mucin spillage, which causes a separation of the epithelium from the connective tissue. The pathologist must be aware of this lesion and should avoid mistaking it microscopically for a vesiculobullous disorder, especially cicatricial (mucous membrane) pemphigoid.

Treatment and Prognosis

Some mucoceles are short-lived lesions that rupture and heal by themselves. Many lesions, however, are chronic in nature, and local surgical excision is necessary. To minimize the risk of recurrence, when the area is excised, the surgeon should remove any adjacent minor salivary glands that may be feeding into the lesion. The excised tissue should be submitted for microscopic examination to conform the diagnosis and rule out the possibility of a salivary gland tumor. The prognosis is excellent, although occasional mucoceles will recur, necessitating reexcision, especially if the feeding glands are not removed

.Mucus Extravasation Cyst

Etiology and Pathogenesis

The cause of mucus extravasation phenomenon is traumatic severance of a salivary gland excretory duct, resulting in mucus escape, or extravasation, into the surrounding connective tissue. An inflammatory reaction of neutrophils followed by macrophages ensues. Granulation tissue forms a wall around the mucin pool, and the contributing salivary gland undergoes inflammatory change. Ultimately, scarring occurs in and around the gland.

Clinical Features

The lower lip is the most common site of mucus extravasation phenomenon, but the buccal mucosa, anterior-ventral surface of the tongue (location of Blandin-Nuhn glands), floor of the mouth, and retromolar region are often affected. Lesions are uncommonly found in other intraoral regions where salivary glands are located, probably because of a lower susceptibility to trauma. Mucus extravasation phenomenon presents as a relatively painless smooth-surfaced mass ranging in size from a few millimeters to 2 cm in diameter. It has a bluish color when mucin is superficially located. Adolescents and children are more commonly affected than adults. Lesions may fluctuate in size because of mucosal rupture over the pooled mucin. Continued production of mucin leads to recurrence. The maximum size is usually reached within several days after injury, and a viscous material is found if aspiration is attempted.

Superficial mucocele

It is a variant of the extravasation-type mucocele. Rather than arising from traumatic duct rupture, this form of mucocele is believed to arise as a result of increased pressure in the outermost part of the excretory duct. These lesions are asymptomatic and numerous, occurring most commonly in the retromolar area, soft palate, and posterior buccal mucosa. Their clinical appearance suggests a vesiculobullous disease, but the lesions persist for an extended time. Other than being a diagnostic challenge, they are of little significance.

Histopathology

Extravasation of free mucin incites an inflammatory response that is followed by connective tissue repair. Neutrophils and macrophages are seen, and granulation tissue forms around the mucin pool. The adjacent salivary gland whose duct was transected shows ductal dilation, chronic inflammation, acinar degeneration, and interstitial fibrosis.

Differential Diagnosis

Although a history of a traumatic event followed by development of a bluish translucency of the lower lip is characteristic of mucus extravasation phenomenon, other lesions might be considered when a typical history is absent. These include salivary gland neoplasm (especially mucoepidermoid carcinoma), vascular malformation, venous varix, and soft tissue neoplasm such as neurofibroma or lipoma. Rarely, a mucocele may appear in the alveolar gingival mucosa. When this is the case, an eruption cyst or gingival cyst should be included in the differential diagnosis.

Treatment and Prognosis

The treatment of mucus extravasation phenomenon is surgical excision. Aspiration of the fluid content provides no lasting clinical benefit. Removal of the associated minor salivary glands along with the pooled mucus is necessary to prevent recurrence.

No treatment is required for superficial mucoceles, since they rupture spontaneously and are short-lived.

Mucus Retention Cyst

Etiology and Pathogenesis

Mucus retention cysts result from obstruction of salivary flow because of a sialolith, periductal scar, or impinging tumor. The retained mucin is surrounded by ductal epithelium, giving the lesion a cyst like appearance microscopically. Obstruction due to a salivary stone, or sialolith, is usually associated with the submandibular gland. The sialolith(s) may be found anywhere in the ductal system from the gland parenchyma to the excretory duct orifice. A sialolith represents the precipitation of calcium salts (predominantly calcium carbonate and calcium phosphate) around a central nidus of cellular debris or inspissated mucin.

Clinical Features

Mucus retention cyst is less common than mucus extravasational phenomenon. It usually appears in an older age-group and is most commonly seen in the upper lip, palate, cheek, and floor of the month. Lesions present as asymptomatic swellings, usually without antecedent trauma. They vary in size from 3 to 10mm and on palpation are mobile and non tender. The overlying mucosa is intact and of normal color. Mucin in floor-of-mouth lesions may penetrate musculature and escape into the soft tissues of the neck, causing a "plunging ranula."

Histopathology

The cystlike cavity of a mucus retention cyst is lined by normal but compressed ductal epithelial cells. The type of lining formed by the epithelial cells ranges from pseudo stratified to stratifiedsquamous. The cyst lumen contains inspissated mucin or a calcified sialolith. The connective tissue around the lesion is minimally inflamed, although the associated gland shows obstructive change.

Differential Diagnosis

Salivary gland neoplasms, mucus extravasation phenomenon, and benign connective-tissue neoplasms should be included in a clinical differential diagnosis. Dermoid cyst might also be included for lesions in the floor of the mouth.

Treatment and Prognosis

Treatment requires removal of the mucus retention cyst and the associated minor salivary gland to avoid postoperative mucus extravasation phenomenon. Lesions of the major salivary glands can be treated in a similar way or, on occasion, only by removal of the obstruction {sialolith} if it occurs in the distal part of the ductal system. The sialolith is either surgically removed or milked through the duct orifice. If a duct is surgically entered, special precautions are used to aid the healing process so that duct scarring is minimized. Constriction of the duct through excessive scar formation could result in recurrence. Marsupialization by the placement of a silk suture in the roof of a large mucus retention cyst, particularly in one arising in the floor of the mouth, can be useful to reduce its size before surgical excision.

RANULAS

A ranula is a large mucocele located on the floor of the mouth. Ranulas may be either mucous extravasation phenomena or mucous extravasation phenomenon involving the lower lip.

With time, fibrosis occurs, replacing the acinar functional cells with connective tissues. The inflammatory components disappear, and a sessile, firm mass is observed on the lower lip with normal mucous membrane. Mucous retention cysts and are most commonly associated with the sublingual salivary gland duct

Etiology

The most common cause of ranula formation is trauma. Other causes include an obstructed salivary gland or a ductal aneurysm. A sarcoid-associated ranula also has been reported.

Clinical Presentation

The term "ranula" is used because this lesion often resembles the swollen abdomen of a frog. The lesion most commonly presents as a painless, slow growing, soft, and movable mass located in the floor of the mouth. Usually, the lesion forms to one side of the lingual frenum; however, if the lesion extends deep into the soft tissue, it can cross the midline. Like mucoceles, superficial ranulas can have a typical bluish hue, but when the lesion is deeply seated, the mucosa may have a normal appearance. The size of the lesions can vary, and larger lesions can cause deviation of the tongue. A deep lesion that herniates through the mylohyoid muscle and extends along the fascial planes is referred to as a plunging ranula and

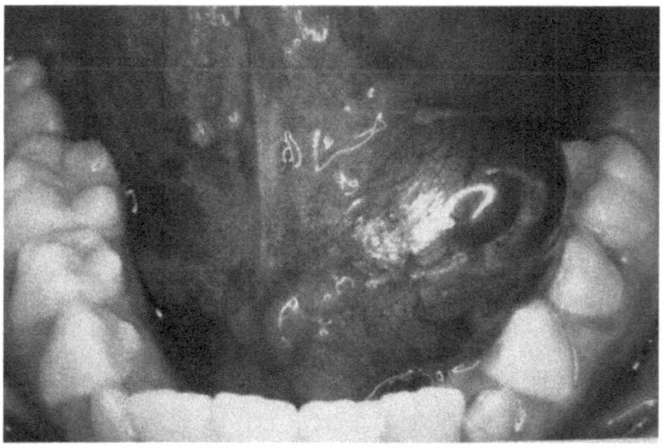

may become large, extending into the neck. Radiography should be performed to rule out a sialolith as a cause of duct obstruction. Radiopaque material instilled into the ranula cavity may be helpful in delineating the borders and full extent of the lesion.

Histopathologic Features

The microscopic appearance of a ranula is similar to that of a mucocele in other locations. The spilled mucin elicits a granulation tissue response that typically contains foamy histiocytes.

Treatment

Ranulas are usually treated sugically. A marsupialization procedure that unroofs the lesion is the initial treatment of choice, especially for smaller lesions. Recurrences have been noted with the marsupialization technique alone, and in these cases, excision of the lesion (including the gland) is recommended. Intralesional injections of corticosteroids have been used succsessfully in the treatment of ranulas.

SALIVARY DUCT CYST (MUCUS RETENTION CYST; MUCUS DUCT CYST; SIALOCYST)

The salivary duct cyst is an epithelium-lined cavity that arises from salivary gland tissue. Unlike the more common mucocele, it is a true cyst because it is lined by epithelium. The cause of such cysts is uncertain. Some cases may represent ductal dilatation secondary to ductal obstruction (e.g., mucus plug which creates increased intraluminal pressure; some authors refer to such lesions as mucus retention cysts .Other cases appear to represent true developmental salivary duct cysts that are separate from the adjacent normal salivary ducts.

Clinical features

Salivary duct cysts usually occur in adults and can arise within either the major or minor glands. Cysts of the major glands are most common within the parotid gland, presenting as slowly growing, asymptomatic swellings Intraoral cysts can occur at any minor gland site, but most frequently they develop in the floor of the mouth, buccal mucosa, and lips. They often look like mucocele and are characterized by a soft, fluctuant swelling that may appear bluish, depending on the depth of the cyst below the surface. Some cysts may feel relatively firm to palpation. Cysts in the floor of the mouth often arise adjacent to the submandibular duct and sometimes have an amber color.

On rare occasions, patients have been observed to develop multiple mucus retention cysts that involve the excretory ducts of many of the minor salivary glands throughout the mouth. The individual lesions often present as painful nodules that demonstrate dilated ductal orifices on the mucosal surface. Mucus or pus may be expressed from these dilated ducts.

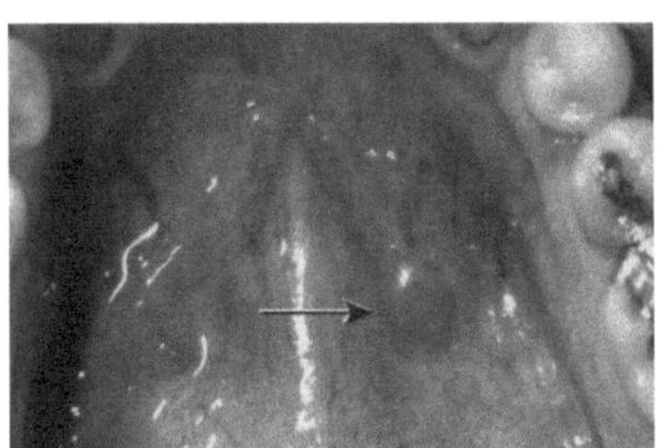

Histopathologic Features

The lining of the salivary duct cyst is variable and may consist of cuboidal, columnar, or atrophic squamous epithelium surrounding thin or mucoid secretions in the lumen. In some cases (especially those caused by ductal obstruction), the epithelium may undergo oncocytic metaplasia, often demonstrating papillary folds into the cystic lumen, somewhat reminiscent of a small Warthin tumor but without the prominent lymphoid stroma. If this proliferation is extensive enough, these lesions are sometimes diagnosed as papillary cystadenoma, although it seems likely that most are not true neoplasms. The individual lesions of patients with multiple mucus retention cysts also show prominent oncocytic metaplasia of the epithelial lining.

Treatment and Prognosis

Isolated salivary duct cysts are treated by conservative surgical excision. For cysts in the major glands, partial or total removal of the gland may be necessary. The lesion for rare patients who develop multiple mucus retention cysts, local excision may be performed for the more problematic swellings; however, surgical management does not appear feasible or advisable for all of the lesions, which may number as many as 100. In one reported case, systemic erythromycin and chlorhexidine mouth rinses were helpful in relieving pain and reducing drainage of pus. Sialagogues also may be helpful in stimulating salivary flow, thereby preventing the accumulation of inspissated mucus within the dilated excretory ducts.

Maxillary Sinus Retention Cyst/Pseudo cyst

Retention cysts and pseudo cysts involving the lining of the maxillary antrum are common findings in panoramic radiographs. These lesions are discovered incidentally and are of little clinical significance.

Etiology and Pathogenesis

Retention cysts are thought to arise from blockage of an antral seromucous gland, resulting in a ductal epithelium-lined cystic structure filled with mucin. Pseudo cysts are inflammatory in origin and result from fluid accumulation within the sinus membrane. They may be related to infection or allergy. Bacterial toxins, anoxia, or other factors presumably cause leakage of protein into surrounding soft tissue, thus raising the extravascular osmotic pressure with subsequent fluid increase.

Clinical Features

The great majority of these lesions are asymptomatic, although there may be some slight tenderness in the mucobuccal fold or, more rarely, palpable buccal expansion in this region. In panoramic and periapical radiographs, retention cysts and pseudo-cysts of the maxillary sinus are hemispheric, homogeneously opaque, and well delineated. They usually demonstrate an attachment to the floor of the antrum, with size being a function of the anatomic space rather than of duration. Uncommonly these lesions may appear bilaterally.

Histopathology

The pathogenesis of the two forms of antral cysts is reflected in the histologic appearance. The retention cyst is lined by pseudo stratified columnar epithelium with occasional mucous cells interspersed. The supportive elements are minimally inflamed. The pseudo cyst shows no evidence of an epithelial lining but, rather, pools of mucoid material surrounded by slightly compressed connective tissue.

Differential Diagnosis

A clinical differential diagnosis of cysts and pseudo cysts arising within the mucosa of the maxillary sinus would include polyps, hyperplasia of the sinus lining secondary to odontogenic infection, maxillary sinusitis, and neoplasms arising within the soft tissues of the antral lining.

Treatment

Antral retention cysts and pseudo cysts are generally left untreated because they are limited in growth and are not destructive, and most spontaneously rupture. Therefore periodic observation is all that is required.

NECROTIZINC SIALOMETAPLASIA

Necrotizing sialometaplasia is an uncommon, locally destructive inflammatory condition of the salivary glands. Although the cause is uncertain, most authors believe it is the result of ischemia of the salivary tissue that leads to local infarction. The importance of this lesion rests in the fact that it mimics a malignant process, both clinically and microscopically. Unnecessary surgery has been performed because of an erroneous preoperative diagnosis of squamous cell carcinoma or mucoepidermoid carcinoma.

Etiology and Pathogenesis

The initiating event of necrotizing sialometaplasia is believed to be salivary gland ischemia precipitated by local trauma, surgical manipulation, or local anesthesia. Infarction of the gland follows, and squamous metaplasia of ductal remnants eventually appears. This condition is believed to be due to local trauma or focal vascular compromise leading to discrete tissue necrosis in the area. Patients often have no history of a prior traumatic event.

A number of potential predisposing factors have been suggested, including the following:

1. Traumatic injuries
2. Dental injections
3. Ill-fitting dentures
4. Upper respiratory infections
5. Adjacent tumors
6. Previous surgery

It has been suggested that these factors may play a role in compromising the blood supply to the involved glands, resulting in ischemic necrosis. However, many cases occur without any known predisposing factors.

Clinical Features

Necrotizing sialometaplasia most frequently develops in the palatal salivary glands; more than 75% of all cases occur on the posterior palate. The hard palate is affected more often than the soft palate. About two thirds of palatal cases are unilateral, with the rest being bilateral or midline in location. Necrotizing sialometaplasia also has been reported in other minor salivary gland sites and, occasionally, in the parotid gland. The submandibular and sublingual glands are rarely affected. Although it can occur at almost any age, necrotizing sialometaplasia is most common in adults; the mean age of onset is 46 years. Males are affected nearly twice as often as females.

The condition appears initially as a nonulcerated swelling, often associated with pain or paresthesia. Within 2 to 3 weeks, necrotic tissue sloughs out, leaving a craterlike ulcer that can range from less than 1 cm to more than 5 cm in diameter. The patient may report that "a part of my palate fell out." At this point, the pain often subsides. In rare instances, there can be destruction of the underlying palatal bone.

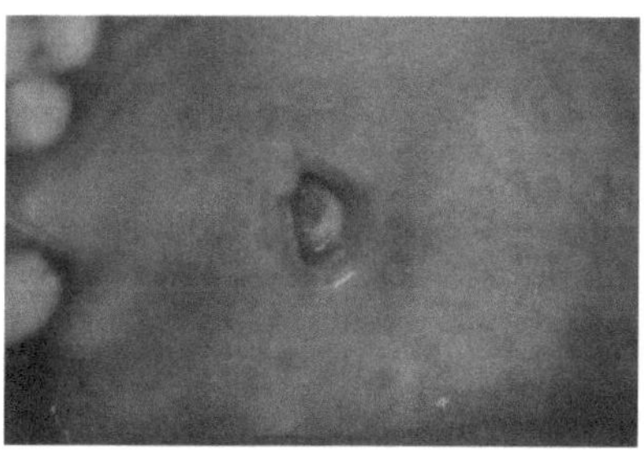

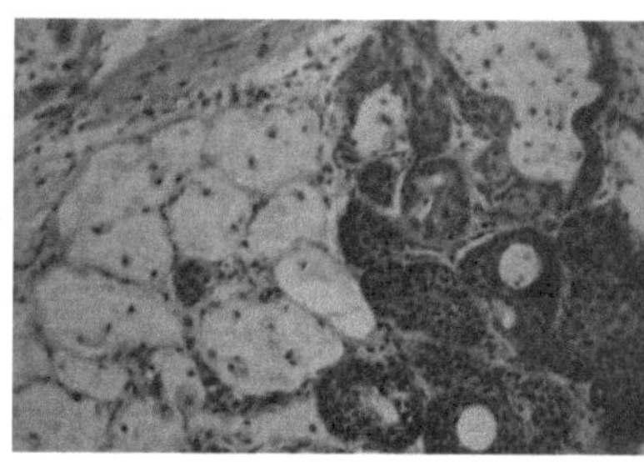

Histopathologic Features

The microscopic appearance of necrotizing sialometaplasia is characterized by acinar necrosis in early lesions, followed by associated squamous metaplasia of the salivary ducts. Although the mucous acinar cells are necrotic, the overall lobular architecture of the involved glands is still preserved—a helpful histopathologic clue. There may be liberation of mucin, with an associated inflammatory response. The squamous metaplasia of the salivary ducts can be striking and produce a pattern that is easily misdiagnosed as squamous cell carcinoma or mucoepidermoid carcinoma. This mistaken impression may be further compounded by the frequent association of pseudoepitheliomatous hyperplasia of the overlying epithelium, in most cases; however, the squamous proliferation has a bland cytologic appearance.

Differential Diagnosis

Clinically, squamous cell carcinoma and malignant minor salivary gland neoplasms must be ruled out, usually by a biopsy. Syphilitic gummas and deep fungal infections must likewise be ruled out, since they may present as punched-out lesions of the palate. Findings from serology, biopsy, and/or culture are usually needed to exclude these entities. In medically compromised patients, such as those with poorly controlled diabetes, opportunistic fungal infections such as mucormycosis may cause a similar clinical picture. The entity subacute necrotizing sialadenitis has recently been described as a nonspecific, inflammatory condition of minor salivary glands of unknown etiology. It is characterized by an abrupt onset of pain and localized swelling, usually of the hard or soft palate, but unlike necrotizing sialometaplasia, is self-limiting without an ulcerative or metaplastic component.

Treatment and Prognosis

Because of the worrisome clinical presentation of necrotizing sialometaplasia, biopsy usually is indicated to rule out the possibility of malignant disease. Once the diagnosis has been established, no specific treatment is indicated or necessary. The lesion typically resolves on its own accord, with an average healing time of 5 to 6 week.

Treatment

It is important for the clinician to understand the etiology and biologic behavior of this lesion and for the pathologist to have expertise on oral lesions. In addition to the specimen, a complete clinical history should be provided to the pathologist to aid in distinguishing this lesion from squamous cell carcinoma. An adequate biopsy specimen is essential since the histologic features of this lesion are unique. Necrosis of the salivary gland, pseudoepitheliomatous hyperplasia of the mucosal epithelium, and squamous metaplasia of the salivary ducts are seen. Histopathologic examination will reveal that there are no malignant cells and that the lobular architecture is preserved even though necrosis is present. Necrotizing sialometaplasia is self-limiting, lasts approximately 6 weeks, and heals by secondary intention. No specific treatment is required, but débridement and saline rinses may help the healing process. Recurrence and impairment are not usually encountered.

SIALORRHEA

Sialorrhea, or excessive salivation, is an uncommon condition that has various causes. Minor sialorrhea may result from local irritations, such as aphthous ulcers or ill-fitting dentures. Patients with new dentures often experience excess saliva production until they become accustomed to the prosthesis. Episodic hyper secretion of saliva, or "water brash," may occur as a protective buffering system to neutralize stomach acid in individuals with gastro esophageal reflux disease. Sialorrhea is a well-known clinical feature of rabies and heavy metal poisoning. It also may occur as a consequence of certain medications, such as lithium and cholinergic agonists. Drooling can be a problem for patients who are mentally retarded, who have a neurologic disorder such as cerebral palsy, or who have undergone surgical resection of the mandible. In these instances, the drooling is probably not caused by overproduction of saliva but due to poor neuromuscular control.

Clinical Features

The excess saliva production typically produces drooling and choking, which may cause social embarrassment. In children with mental retardation or cerebral palsy, the uncontrolled salivary flow may lead to macerated sores around the mouth, chin, and neck that can become secondarily infected. The constant soiling of clothes and bed linens can be a significant problem for the parents and caretakers of these patients.

An interesting type of super salivation of unknown cause has been termed idiopathic paroxysmal sialorrhea. Individuals with this condition experience short episodes of excessive salivation lasting from 2 to 5 minutes. These episodes are associated with a prodrome of nausea or epigastric pain.

Treatment and Prognosis

Some causes of sialorrhea are transitory or mild, and no treatment is needed. For individuals with increased salivation associated with gastro esophageal reflux disease, medical management of their reflux problem may be beneficial. For persistent severe drooling, therapeutic intervention may be indicated. Anticholinergic medications can decrease saliva production but may produce unacceptable side effects. Transdermal scopolamine has been tried with some success, but it should not be used in children younger than age 10. Speech therapy can be used to improve neuromuscular control, but patient cooperation is necessary.

Several surgical techniques have been used successfully to control severe drooling in individuals with poor neuromuscular control:

* Relocation of the submandibular ducts (sometimes along with excision of the sublingual glands)

• Relocation of the parotid ducts

* Submandibular gland excision plus parotid duct ligation

* Bilateral tympanic neurectomy with sectioning of the chorda tympani

In ductal relocation, the ducts are repositioned posteriorly to the tonsillar fossa, thereby redirecting salivary flow and minimizing drooling. The use of bilateral tympanic neurectomy and sectioning of the chorda tympani destroys parasympathetic innervation to the glands, reducing salivary secretions and possibly inducing xerostomia. However, this procedure also produces a loss of taste to the anterior two thirds of the tongue.

XEROSTOMIA

Xerostomia refers to a subjective sensation of a dry mouth; it is frequently, but not always, associated with salivary gland hypo function. A number of factors play a role in the cause of xerostomia; Xerostomia is a common problem that has been reported in 25% of older adults. In the past, complaints of dry mouth in older patients often were ascribed to the predictable result of aging. However, it is now generally accepted that any reductions in salivary function associated with age are modest and probably are not associated with any significant reduction in salivary function. Instead, xerostomia in older adults is more likely to be the result of other factors, especially medications. 500 drugs have been reported to produce xerostomia as a side effect, including 63% of the 200 most frequently prescribed medicines in the United States. Not only are specific drugs known to produce dry mouth, but the prevalence of xerostomia also increases in relation to the total number of drugs that a person takes, regardless whether the individual medications are xerogenic or not.

Causes of Xerostomia

DEVELOPMENTAL

Salivary gland aplasia

WATER/METABOLITE LOSS

Impaired fluid intake

Hemorrhage

Vomiting/diarrhea

IATROCENIC

Medications

Radiation therapy to the head and neck

SYSTEMIC DISEASES

Sjogren syndrome

Diabetes mellitus

Diabetes insipidus

Sarcoidosis

HIV infection

Craft versus-host disease

Psychogenic disorders

LOCAL FACTORS

Decreased mastication

Smoking

Mouth breathing

Medications that May Produce Xerostomia

CLASS OF DRUG	EXAMPLE
Antihistamines	Diphenhydramine Chlorpheniramine
Decongestartts	Pseudoephedrine
Antidepressants	Amitriptyline
Antipsychotic	Phenothiazine derivatives Haloperidol
Antihypertensives	Reserpine Methyldopa Chiorothiazide Furosemide Metoprolol Calcium channel blockers
Anticholinergics	Atropine Scopolamine

Clinical Features

Examination of the patient typically demonstrates a reduction in salivary secretions, and the residual appears cither foamy or thick and "ropey." The mucosa appears dry and the clinician may notice that the examining gloves stick to the mucosal surfaces. The dorsal tongue often is fissured with atrophy of the filiform papillae. The patient may complain of difficulty with mastication and swallowing and may even indicate that food adheres to the oral membranes during eating. The clinical findings, however, do not always correspond to the patient's symptoms. Some patients who complain of dry mouth may appear to have adequate salivary flow and oral moistness. Conversely, some patients who clinically appear to have a dry mouth have no complaints. The degree of saliva production can be assessed by measuring both resting and stimulated salivary flow.

There is an increased prevalence of oral candidiasis in patients with xerostomia because of the reduction in the cleansing and antimicrobial activity normally provided by saliva. In addition, these patients are more prone to dental decay, especially cervical and root caries. This problem has been associated more often with radiation therapy, and it is some times called radiation induced caries but more appropriately should be called xerostomia-related caries

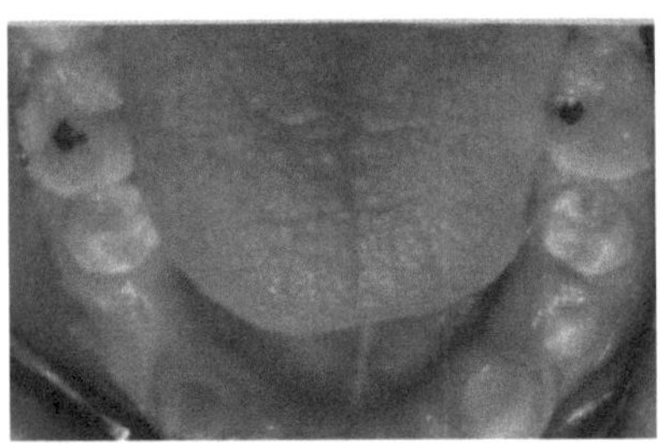

TREATMENT OF XEROSTOMIA

Treatment that is available for the dry mouth patient can be divided into four main categories:

(1) Preventive therapy,

(2) Symptomatic treatment,

(3) Local or topical salivary stimulation, and

(4) Systemic salivary stimulation.

Effective treatment of an underlying systemic disorder associated with salivary gland dysfunction may correct the salivary complaint as well.

Preventive Therapy

The use of topical fluorides in a patient with salivary gland hypo function is absolutely critical to control dental caries. There are many different fluoride therapies available (eg, over-the counter fluoride rinses, brush-on forms, and highly concentrated prescription fluorides that can be applied by brush or in a custom carrier). The frequency of application (from daily to once per week) should be modified, depending on the severity of the salivary dysfunction and the rate of caries development. It is essential that patients maintain meticulous oral hygiene. Patients will require more frequent dental visits (usually every 4 months) and must work closely with the dentist to maintain good dental health. When salivary function is compromised, there may be an increase in demineralization, speeding the loss of tooth structure. Remineralizing solutions may be used to alleviate some of the effects of the loss of normal salivation. Patients with dry mouth also experience an increase in oral infections, particularly mucosal candidiasis. This may take an erythematous form (without the easily recognized pseudo membranous plaques), and the patient may present with redness of the mucosa and complains of a burning sensation of the tongue or other intraoral soft tissues. A high index of suspicion should be maintained, and appropriate antifungal therapies should be instituted as necessary. Patients with salivary gland dysfunction may require prolonged treatment periods and re-treatment to eradicate oral fungal infections.

Symptomatic Treatment

Several symptomatic treatments are available. Water is by far the most important. Patients should be encouraged to sip water throughout the day; this will help to moisten the oral cavity, hydrate the mucosa, and clear debris from the mouth. The use of water with meals can make chewing and forming the food bolus easier, will ease swallowing, and will improve taste perception. An increase in environmental humidity is exceedingly important. The use of room humidifiers, particularly at night, may lessen discomfort markedly. As part of the normal diurnal variation, salivary flow drops almost to zero during rest. In individuals who have any degree of secretory hypo function, the dessication of the mucosa is particularly troublesome at night and may interfere with restorative sleep. There are a number of oral rinses and gels available. Patients should be cautioned to avoid products containing alcohol, sugar, or strong flavorings that may irritate sensitive dry mucosa .Moisturizing creams are important. The frequent use of products containing aloe vera or vitamin E should be encouraged. Persistent cracking and erythema at the corners of the mouth should be investigated for a fungal cause.

There are many commercially available salivary substitutes. However, saliva replacements (artificial salvias) are not well accepted by most patients. While there is clearly a role for the use of saliva replacements, particularly in individuals who have no residual salivary gland function, it must be recognized that this is not a highly effective symptomatic therapy.

Salivary Stimulation

LOCAL OR TOPICAL STIMULATION

Several approaches are available for stimulating salivary flow. Chewing will stimulate salivary flow effectively, as will sour and sweet tastes. The combination of chewing and taste, as provided by gums or mints, can be very effective in relieving symptoms for patients who have remaining salivary function. Patients with dry mouth must be told not to use products that contain sugar as a sweetener, due to the increased risk for dental caries in this group. Electrical stimulation has also been used as a therapy for salivary hypo function but has been inadequately investigated clinically. A device that delivers a very low- voltage electrical charge to the tongue and palate has been described although its effect was modest in patients with dry mouth.

SYSTEMIC STIMULATION

The use of systemic secretogogues for salivary stimulation has also been examined, with mixed results. More than 24 agents have been proposed as means of stimulating salivary output systemically. Four have been examined extensively in controlled clinical trials; these are bromhexine, anetholetrithione, pilocarpine hydrochloride, and cevimeline hydrochloride. Bromhexine is a mucolytic agent used in Europe and the Middle East. The proposed mechanism of action for salivary stimulation is unknown. No proven benefit to salivary function has been shown by objective and controlled clinical trials. Bromhexine may stimulate lacrimal function in patients with Sjögren's syndrome although this is controversial. Anetholetrithione is a mucolytic agent that has been shown to increase salivary output in clinical trials. The mechanism of action is not definitively known, but it has been suggested that anetholetrithione may up-regulate muscarinic receptors. In patients with mild salivary gland hypo function, anetholetrithione significantly increased saliva flow. However, it was ineffective in patients with marked salivary gland hypo function. The adverse effects are mild. One study suggested a possible synergistic effect of anetholetrithione in combination with pilocarpine. Pilocarpine hydrochloride is approved specifically for the relief of xerostomia. Current indications are for patients with dryness following radiotherapy for head and neck cancers and for those with Sjögren's syndrome. Pilocarpine HCL is a parasympathomimetic drug, functioning as a muscarinic cholinergic agonist. Pilocarpine increases salivary output, stimulating any remaining gland function. The adverse effects of pilocarpine in human studies are very common and are usually mild. They are consistent with the known mechanism of action of the drug. Sweating is the most common side effect. Other frequently reported side effects are hot flashes, urinary frequency, diarrhea, and blurred vision.

After the administration of pilocarpine, salivary output increases fairly rapidly, usually reaching a maximum within 1 hour. The best-tolerated doses are those of 5.0 to 7.5 mg, given three or four times daily. The duration of action is approximately 2 to 3 hours. Pilocarpine is contraindicated for patients with pulmonary disease, asthma, cardiovascular disease, glaucoma, or urethral reflux. Patients do not appear to develop tolerance to pilocarpine following prolonged use. Pilocarpine has been shown to be a safe and effective therapy for patients with diminished salivation but who have some remaining secretory function that can be stimulated. Cevimeline HCl is another parasympathomimetic agonist that has been recently approved for the treatment of symptoms of oral dryness in Sjögren's syndrome. This medication reportedly specifically targets the muscarinic receptors of the salivary and lacrimal glands. It still must be used with caution in patients with a history of glaucoma or cardiovascular, respiratory, or gall bladder disease and in patients who use various medications. Its side effects are similar to those of pilocarpine. To date, there have been few published reports of clinical trials with cevimeline.

Pilocarpine HCl and cevimeline HCl are the only systemic sialagogues that are available in the United States. Medical consultation prior to prescribing these drugs for patients with significant medical conditions may be indicated. Increased understanding of the causes of xerostomia and salivary gland hypo function undoubtedly will lead to improvement in the available treatments through the design and testing of more rational and specific therapies.

Salivary gland tumors

GENERAL CONSIDERATIONS

Tumors of the salivary glands constitute an important area in the field of oral and maxillofacial pathology. Although such tumors are uncommon, they are by no means rare. The annual incidence of salivary gland tumors around the world ranges from about 1 to 6.5 cases per 100,000 people. Although soft tissue neoplasms (e.g., hemangioma), lymphoma, and metastatic tumors can occur within the salivary glands, the discussion in this chapter is limited to primary epithelial neoplasms,

An often-bewildering array of different salivary tumors have been identified and categorized. In addition, the classification scheme is a dynamic one that changes as clinicians learn more about these lesions. A number of investigators have published their findings on salivary gland neoplasia, but a comparison of these studies is often difficult. Some studies have been limited to only the major glands or have not included all the minor salivary gland sites. In addition, the ever-evolving classification system makes an evaluation of some older studies difficult, especially when we try to compare them with more recent analyses. Not withstanding these difficulties, it is still helpful to compare these studies because they provide a good overview of salivary neoplasia in general. An evaluation of various studies shows fairly consistent trends (with minor variations) with regard to salivary gland tumors.

Classification of Salivary Gland Tumors

BENIGN

1. Pleomorphic adenoma (mixed tumor)
2. Myoepithelioma
3. Basal cell adenoma
4. Canalicular adenoma
5. Warthin tumor (papillary cystadenoma lymphomatosum)
6. Oncocytoma
7. Sebaceous adenoma
8. Sebaceous lymph adenoma
9. Ductal papillomas
10. Sialadenoma papilliferurn
11. Intraductal papilloma
12. Inverted ductal papilloma
13. Papillary cystadenoma
14. Sialoblastoma

MALIGNANT

1. Malignant mixed tumors
2. Carcinoma ex pleomorphic adenoma
3. Sarcoma
4. Metastasizing mixed tumor
5. Mucoepidermoid carcinoma
6. Acinic cell adenocarcinoma
7. Adenoid cystic carcinoma
8. Polymorphous low-grade adenocarcinoma

9. Basal cell adenocarcinoma
10. Epithelial-myoepithelial Carcinoma
11. Salivary duct carcinoma
12. Myoepithelial carcinoma
13. Cystadenocarcinoma
14. Sebaceous adenocarcinoma
15. Sebaceous lymph adenocarcinoma
16. Clear cell adenocarcinoma
17. Oncocytic carcinoma
18. Squamous cell carcinoma
19. Malignant lymphoepithelial lesion (lymphoepithelial carcinoma)
20. Small cell carcinoma
21. Adenocarcinoma, not otherwise specified (NOS)

The most common site for salivary gland tumors is the parotid gland, accounting for 64% to 80% of all cases. Fortunately, a relatively low percentage of parotid tumors are malignant, ranging from 15% to 32%. Overall, it can be stated that two thirds to three quarters of all salivary tumors occur in the parotid, and two thirds to three quarters of these parotid tumors are benign.

The pleomorphic adenoma is overwhelmingly the most common tumor (53% to 77% of all cases in the parotid gland). Warthin tumors are also fairly common; they account for 6% to 14% of cases. A variety of malignant tumors occur, with the mucoepidermoid carcinoma appearing to be the most frequent overall. However, two studies from Great Britain show a significantly lower prevalence of this tumor, possibly indicative of a geographic difference, especially compared with reports of cases from the United States.
From 8% to 11% of all salivary tumors occur in the submandibular gland, but the frequency of malignancy in this gland is almost double that of the parotid gland, ranging from 37% to 45%. However, as shown in Table 11-5, the pleomorphic adenoma is still the most common tumor and makes up 44% to 68% of all neoplasms. Unlike its occurrence in the parotid gland, the Warthin tumor is unusual in the submandibular gland, making up no more than 1% to 2% of all tumors. Adenoid cystic carcinoma is the most common malignancy, ranging from 12% to 27% of all cases. Tumors of the sublingual gland are rare, comprising no more than 1% of all salivary neoplasms. However, 70% to 90% of sublingual tumors are malignant.

Tumors of the various smaller minor salivary glands make up 9% to 23% of all tumors, which makes this group the second most common site for salivary neoplasia .Unfortunately, a relatively high proportion (almost 50%) of these have been malignant in most studies. Excluding rare sublingual tumors, it can be stated that the smaller the gland, the greater the likelihood of malignancy for a salivary gland tumor.

As observed in the major glands, the pleomorphic adenoma is the most common minor gland tumor and accounts for about 40% of all cases. The mucoepidermoid carcinoma and adenoid cystic carcinoma generally have been considered the two most common malignancies, although the recently delineated polymorphous low-grade adenocarcinoma also is becoming recognized as one of the more common minor gland tumors.

The palate is the most frequent site for minor salivary gland tumors, with 42% to 54% of all cases found there. Most of these occur on the posterior lateral hard or soft palate, which have the greatest concentration of glands. The lips are the second most common location for minor gland tumors (21 % to 22% of cases), followed by the buccal mucosa (11 % to 15% of cases). Labial tumors are significantly more common in the upper lip, which accounts for 77% to 89% of all lip tumors although mucoceles are commonly found on the lower lip; this is a surprisingly rare site for salivary gland tumors.

Significant differences in the percentage of malignancies and the relative frequency of various tumors can be noted for different minor salivary gland sites. 42% to 50% of tumors of the palate and buccal mucosa sites are malignant, similar to the overall prevalence of malignancy in all minor salivary gland sites combined. In the upper lip, however, only 14% to 25% of tumors are malignant because of the high prevalence of the Canalicular adenoma, which has a special affinity for this location. In contrast, although lower lip tumors are uncommon, 50% to 86% are malignant (mostly mucoepidermoid carcinomas). Up to 91 % of retromolar tumors are malignant, also because of a predominance of mucoepidermoid carcinomas; unfortunately, most tumors in the floor of the mouth and tongue are also malignant

BENIGN NEOPLASMS

At approximately 5 months of embryonic development, a characteristic lobular architecture of salivary glands becomes established. As branching morphogenesis continues, terminal tubular elements give rise to striated intralobular ducts, intercalated ducts, acini, and myoepithelial cells. Intralobular and inter-lobular ducts of the excretory system arise from the remaining progenitor stalk cells. A stem cell or reserve cell within the salivary duct system is believed by many to be the cell of origin of salivary gland neoplasms. Because of their relatively undifferentiated ultra structural appearance, intercalated duct cells are also thought to be capable of giving rise to these neoplasms. The importance of the myoepithelial cell in the composition and growth of numerous epithelial salivary tumors is considerable. Cells with a myoepithelial phenotype can be seen in all salivary gland tumors and are particularly abundant in mixed tumors, myoepitheliomas, adenoid cystic carcinomas, and epimyoepithelial carcinoma of intercalated duct origin.

The three major paired salivary glands—parotid, submandibular, and sublingual—plus the hundreds of small minor salivary glands located within the submucosa of the oral cavity and oropharynx are capable of giving rise to a wide range of neoplasms. The vast majority of salivary neoplasms are epithelial in origin; rarely, the interstitial connective tissue components of the major salivary glands give rise to primary neoplasms whose behavior is similar to that of their extra glandular counterparts. The ratio of benign to malignant salivary gland tumors is gland dependent.

Benign Salivary Gland Tumors

Mixed tumor (pleomorphic adenoma)

Monomorphic adenomas

- Warthin's tumor and papillary cystadenoma sebaceous adenoma
- Oncocytic tumors
- Oncocytoma
- Basal cell adenomas—solid, tubular, trabecular, membranous
- Canalicular adenoma

Myoepithelioma

Ductal papillomas

1. Inverted ductal papilloma
2. Sialadenoma papilliferum
3. Intraductal papilloma

Mixed Tumor (Pleomorphic Adenoma)

The histogenesis of mixed tumor, or pleomorphic adenoma, relates to a dual proliferation of cells with ductal or myoepithelial features, separating it from monomorphic adenomas composed of only one cell type. The myoepithelial-differentiated cell assumes an important role in determining the overall composition and appearance of mixed tumors. A range of cell types and microscopic patterns are seen in mixed tumors—those composed almost completely of epithelial cells at one end of a spectrum and those composed almost completely of myoepithelial cells at the other end. Between these two extremes, less well developed cells with features of both myoepithelial and ductal elements may he seen. Alternatively, it has been theorized that rather than simultaneous proliferation of neoplastic epithelial and myoepithelial cells, a single cell with the potential to differentiate toward either epithelial or myoepithelial cells may be responsible for these tumors. A remarkable microscopic diversity can exist from one tumor to the next, as well as in different areas of the same tumor. The terms pleomorphic adenoma and mixed tumor both represent attempts to describe this tumor's unusual histopathologic features, but neither term is entirely accurate. Although the basic tumor pattern is highly variable, rarely are the individual cells actually pleomorphic. (However, focal minor atypia is acceptable.) Likewise, although the tumor often has a prominent mesenchyme-appearing "stromal" component, it is not truly a mixed neoplasm that is derived from more than one germ layer.

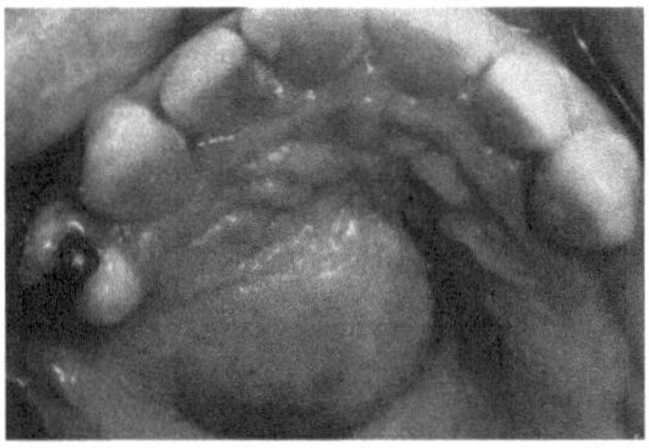

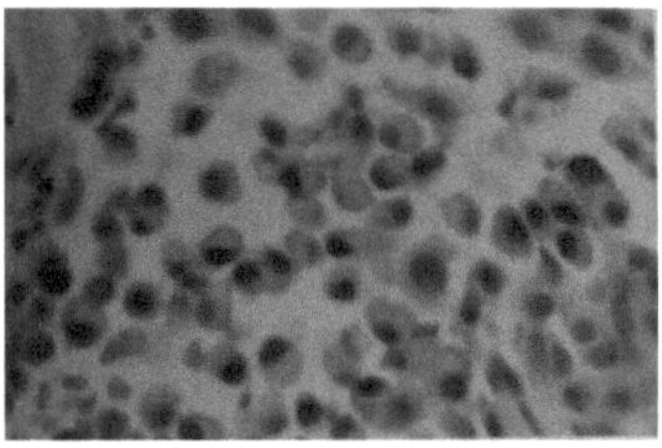

Clinical Features

The mixed tumor, or pleomorphic adenoma, is the most common tumor of the major and minor salivary glands. The parotid gland accounts for approximately 85% of these tumors, whereas the submandibular gland and the intraoral minor salivary glands account for 8% and 7%, respectively. Mixed tumors occur at any age, favor males slightly more than females, and are most prevalent in the fourth through sixth decades of life. They constitute approximately 50% of all intraoral minor salivary gland tumors. Generally, they are mobile except when they occur in the hard palate. They appear as firm, painless swellings and, in the vast majority of cases, do not cause ulceration of the overlying mucosa. The palate is the most common intraoral site, followed by the upper lip and buccal mucosa.

When they arise within the parotid gland, mixed tumors are generally painless and slow growing. They are usually located below the ear and posterior to the mandible. Some tumors may be grooved by the posterior extent of the mandibular ramus, with long-standing lesions capable of producing pressure atrophy on this bone. When they are situated within the inferior pole or tail of the parotid, the tumors may present below the angle of the mandible and anterior to the sternocleidomastoid muscle. Facial nerve palsy and pain are rare. Initially, the tumor is movable but becomes less mobile as it grows larger. If neglected, the lesion can grow to grotesque proportions. About 10% of parotid mixed tumors develop within the deep lobe of the gland beneath the facial nerve. Sometimes these lesions grow in a medial direction between the ascending ramus and stylomandibular ligament, resulting in a dumbbell-shaped tumor that appears as a mass of the lateral pharyngeal wall or soft palate.

The palate is the most common site for minor gland mixed tumors, accounting for approximately 60% of intraoral examples. This is followed by the upper lip (20%) and buccal mucosa (10%). Palatal tumors almost always are found on the posterior lateral aspect of the palate, presenting as smooth-surfaced, dome-shaped masses. If the tumor is traumatized, secondary ulceration may occur. Because of the tightly bound nature of the hard palate mucosa, tumors in this location are not movable, although those in the lip or buccal mucosa frequently are mobile.

Mixed tumors range in size from a few millimeters to several centimeters in diameter and are capable of reaching giant proportions in the major salivary glands, especially the parotid. The tumor is typically lobulated and enclosed within a connective tissue pseudo capsule that varies in thickness. In areas where the capsule is deficient, neoplastic tissue may lie in direct contact with adjacent salivary tissue and may contribute to recurrences.

Histopathologic Features

The pleomorphic adenoma is typically a well-circumscribed, encapsulated tumor. However, the capsule may be incomplete or show infiltration by tumor cells. This lack of complete encapsulation is more common for minor gland tumors, especially along the superficial aspect of palatal tumors beneath the epithelial surface. The tumor is composed of a mixture of glandular epithelium and myoepithelial cells within a mesenchyme-like background. The ratio of the epithelial elements and the mesenchyme-like component is highly variable among different tumors. Some tumors may consist almost entirely of background "stroma." Others are highly cellular with little background alteration.

The epithelium often forms ducts and cystic structures or may occur as islands or sheets of cells. Keratinizing squamous cells and mucus- producing cells also can also be seen.

Myoepithelial cells often make up a large percentage of the tumor cells and have a variable morphology, sometimes appearing angular or spindled. Some myoepithelial cells are rounded and demonstrate an eccentric nucleus and eosinophilic hyalinized cytoplasm, thus resembling plasma cells. These characteristic plasmacytoid myoepithelial cells are more prominent in tumors arising in the minor glands.

The highly characteristic "stromal" changes are believed to be produced by the myoepithelial cells. Extensive accumulation of mucoid material may occur between the tumor cells, resulting in a myxomatous background. Vacuolar degeneration of cells in these areas can produce a chondroid appearance. In many tumors, the stroma exhibits areas of an eosinophilic, hyalinized change. At times, fat or osteoid also is seen.

Occasionally, salivary tumors are seen that are composed almost entirely of myoepithelial cells with no ductal elements. Such tumors often are called myoepitheliomas, although they probably represent one end of the spectrum of mixed tumors.

Treatment and Prognosis

The treatment of choice is surgical excision. Enucleation of parotid mixed tumors is not advisable because of the risk of recurrence due to extension of tumor through capsular defects. Removal of mixed tumors arising within the parotid gland is complicated by the presence of the facial nerve. Any surgical approach, therefore, must include preservation of the uninvolved facial nerve. In most cases superficial parotidectomy (lateral lobectomy) with preservation of the facial nerve is the most appropriate management for those tumors arising within the parotid. Resection of the submandibular gland is the preferred treatment for mixed tumors in this location. Lesions of the palate or gingiva often involve or abut periosteum or bone, making complete removal difficult unless some bone is removed. Other oral benign mixed tumors can be more easily excised, preferably including tissue beyond the pseudo capsule. Inadequate initial removal of mixed tumors in major glands may result in recurrence, often with multiple, discrete tumor foci. These recurrent lesions may be widely distributed within the area of previous surgery and may occur in association with the surgical scar. In most instances the recurrent tumor maintains the original pathology; however, with each recurrence there is an increased possibility of malignant transformation (carcinoma ex-mixed tumor). The proportion of mixed tumors undergoing malignant transformation is not known with certainty, since almost all tumors are treated fairly early in their clinical course. However, if lesions are untreated for an extended length of time, typically years to decades, up to 25% may undergo malignant transformation. The probability of malignant change also increases if the area has previously been treated with surgery or radiotherapy.

MONOMORPHIC ADENOMA

The term monomorphic adenoma was originally used to describe a group of benign salivary gland tumors demonstrating a more uniform histopathologic pattern than the common pleomorphic adenoma. In some classification schemes, a variety of tumors were included under the broad heading of monomorphic adenoma, including Warthin tumor, oncocytoma, basal cell adenoma, and canalicular adenoma. Other authors have used this term more specifically as a synonym just for the basal cell adenoma or canalicular adenoma. Because of its ambiguous nature, the term monomorphic adenoma probably should be avoided, and each of the tumors mentioned should be referred to by its more specific name.

BASAL CELL ADENOMA

The basal cell adenoma is a benign salivary tumor that derives its name from the basaloid appearance of the tumor cells. It is an uncommon neoplasm that represents only 1 % to 2% of all salivary tumors. Because of its uniform histopathologic appearance, it often has been classified as one of the monomorphic adenomas. However, as mentioned previously, this term probably should be avoided because of its imprecise and frequently confusing definition. Also, ultra structural and immunohistochemical studies have shown that basal cell adenomas are not necessarily composed of only one cell type but sometimes of a combination of salivary ductal epithelium and myoepithelial cells. The basal cell adenoma shows some histopathologic similarity to the canalicular adenoma; in the past, these two terms have been used synonymously. However, histopathologic and clinical differences can be noted that warrant that they be considered as distinct entities.

Clinical Features

Unlike the canalicular adenoma, the basal cell adenoma is primarily a tumor of the parotid gland, with around 75% of all cases occurring there. However, the minor glands represent the second most common site, specifically the glands of the upper lip and buccal mucosa. The tumor can occur at any age but is most common in middle-aged and older adults, with peak prevalence in the seventh decade of life. The tumor appears to be more common in females, with some studies showing as high as a 2:1 female-to-male ratio.

Clinically, the basal cell adenoma appears as a slowly growing, freely movable mass similar to a pleomorphic lobe of the gland. Most tumors are less than 3 cm in diameter. Parotid tumors are located within the superficial lobe of the gland. One subtype, the membranous basal cell adenoma, deserves separate mention. This form of the tumor appears to be hereditary, often occurring in combination with skin appendage tumors, such as dermal cylindromas and trichoepitheliomas. Multiple bilateral tumors may develop within the parotids. Because these tumors often bear a histopathologic resemblance to the skin tumors, they also have been called dermal analogue tumors

Histopathologic Features

The basal cell adenoma is usually encapsulated or well circumscribed. The most common subtype is the solid variant, which consists of multiple islands and cords of epithelial cells that are supported by a small amount of fibrous stroma. The peripheral cells of these islands are palisaded and cuboidal to columnar in shape, similar to the microscopic appearance of basal cell carcinoma. These peripheral cells are frequently hyperchromatic; the central cells of the islands tend to have paler staining nuclei. The central cells occasionally form eddies or keratin pearls.

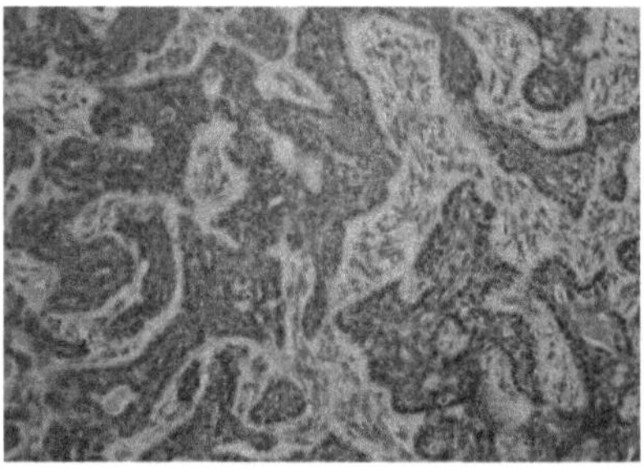

The trabecular subtype demonstrates narrow cordlike epithelial strands. The tubular subtype is characterized by the formation of small, round, duct like structures. Frequently, a mixture of histopathologic subtypes is seen.

The membranous basal cell adenoma exhibits multiple large lobular islands of tumor that are molded together in a jigsaw puzzle fashion. These islands are surrounded by a thick layer of hyaline material, which represents reduplicated basement membrane. Similar hyaline droplets also are often found among the epithelial cells. The microscopic appearance is similar to that of a dermal cylindroma, one of the skin tumors with which it is often associated.

Treatment and Prognosis

The treatment of basal cell adenoma is similar to that of pleomorphic adenoma and consists of complete surgical removal. Recurrence is rare for most histopathologic subtypes. However, the membranous subtype has a 25% to 37% recurrence rate, possibly related to its multifocal nature. The malignant counterpart of the basal cell adenoma is the basal cell adenocarcinoma. Most basal cell adenocarcinomas arise de novo, but some examples from malignant degeneration of a preexisting basal adenoma. Fortunately, these tumors have a relatively good prognosis; although local recurrence is common, the tumor rarely metastasizes or results in death.

CANALICULAR ADENOMA

The canalicular adenoma is an uncommon tumor that occurs almost exclusively in the minor salivary glands. Because of its uniform microscopic pattern, the canalicular adenoma also has been called a "monomorphic adenoma" However, because this term also has been applied to other tumors, its use probably should be discontinued. Likewise, the term basal cell adenoma some-times has been used synonymously for this tumor but should be avoided because it refers to a separate tumor with different clinical features

Clinical Features

The canalicular adenoma shows a striking predilection for the upper lip, with nearly 75% occurring in this location. It represents the first or second most common tumor (along with pleomorphic adenoma) of the upper lip. The buccal mucosa is the second most common site. Occurrence in other minor salivary glands is uncommon, and canalicular adenomas of the parotid gland are rare.

The tumor nearly always occurs in older adults, with peak prevalence in the seventh decade of life. There is a definite female predominance, ranging from 1.2 to 1.8 females for each male.

The canalicular adenoma appears as a slowly growing, painless mass that usually ranges from several millimeters to 2 cm. It may be firm or somewhat fluctuant to palpation. The overlying mucosa may be normal in color or bluish and can be mistaken for a mucocele. However, mucoceles of the upper lip are rare. In some instances, the lesion has been noted to be multifocal, with multiple separate tumors discovered in the upper lip or buccal mucosa.

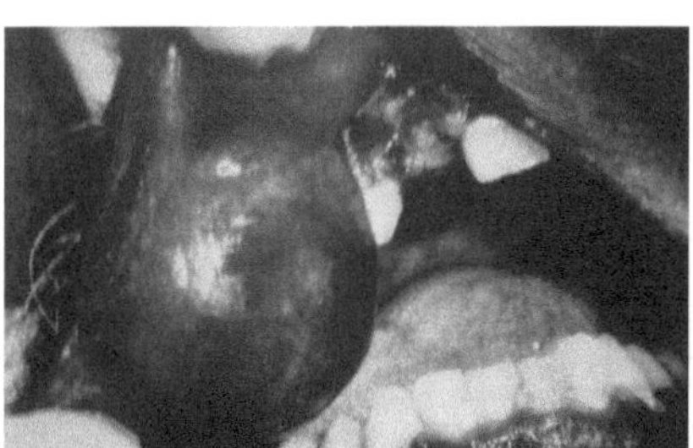

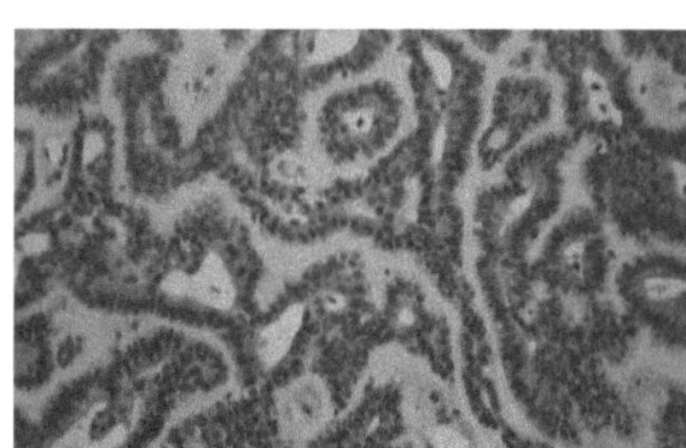

Histopathologic Features

The microscopic pattern of canalicular adenoma is monomorphic in nature. This pattern is characterized by single-layered cords of columnar or cuboidal epithelial cells with deeply basophilic nuclei. In some areas, adjacent parallel rows of cells may be seen, resulting in a bilayered appearance of the tumor cords. These cells enclose ductal structures, sometimes in the form of long canals. Larger cystic spaces often are created, and the epithelium may demonstrate papillary projections into the cystic lumina. The tumor cells are supported by a loose connective tissue stroma with prominent vascularity. Unlike the appearance in pleomorphic adenomas, stromal alterations, such as chon-droid metaplasia, do not occur. A thin, fibrous capsule often surrounds the tumor, although incipient foci of additional tumors sometimes are observed in the surrounding salivary gland tissue.

Treatment and Prognosis

The canalicular adenoma is best treated by local surgical excision. Recurrence is uncommon and actually may represent cases that are multifocal in nature.

Myoepitheliomas

Benign salivary gland tumors composed entirely of myoepithelial cells are called myoepitheliomas. Although these tumors are of epithelial origin, the phenotypic expression of the tumor cells is more closely related to that of smooth muscle. Reflective of this is the immunohistochemical staining of myoepitheliomas cells with antibodies to actins, cytokeratin, and S-100 protein. Most myoepitheliomas arise within the parotid gland and, less commonly, the submandibular gland and intraoral minor salivary glands.

Clinical features

Clinically, myoepitheliomas present as circumscribed painless masses. Lesions appear from the third through ninth decades (median age, 53 years) and in both genders equally.

Histologic features

Microscopically, sheets of either plasmacytoid or spindle cells make up these lesions. Approximately 70% of cases contain spindle cells, and approximately 20% are composed of plasmacytoid cells. Occasionally, both cell forms may be seen in approximately equal quan-tity. Myoepithelial differentiation of tumor cells has been confirmed with immunohistochemical and electron microscopic studies. Rarely, clear cells may dominate the histologic presentation, leading to the designation of a "clear cell variant" of this entity.

Treatment

Treatment of this benign lesion is identical to that of the benign mixed tumor. Conservative excision of lesions arising in minor salivary glands is advised, including a thin rim of surrounding normal tissue. When lesions are noted within the parotid gland, superficial parotidectomy is indicated. The overall prognosis is excellent, and recurrences are not expected.

ONCOCYTOMA

Oncocytomas are less common benign tumors that make up less than 1% of all salivary gland neoplasms. The name of the tumor is derived from the fact that it contains oncocytes, which are large granular acidophilic cells. This tumor occurs almost exclusively in the parotid glands and is equally distributed in both men and women. The sixth decade is the most common time of presentation.

Clinical Presentation

Oncocytomas are usually solid round tumors that can be seen in any of the major salivary glands but that are extremely rare intraorally. These lesions can be found commonly in the superficial lobe of the parotid gland. Bilateral presentation of this tumor can occur, and it is the second most common salivary gland tumor that occurs bilaterally (after Warthin's tumor).

Pathology

On gross examination, these tumors appear noncystic and firm. Histologically, they consist of brown granular eosinophilic cells. The oncocytes within this tumor concentrate technetium, and this tumor can be visualized by Tc-99m Scintigraphy .Malignant oncocytomas can occur, and these are aggressive lesions.

Treatment

Oncocytomas demonstrate a very slow growth rate and a benign course. Superficial parotidectomy with preservation of the facial nerve is the treatment of choice for parotid gland tumors. Removal of the gland is the treatment of choice for tumors in the submandibular gland, and gland removal with a normal cuff of tissue is the treatment of choice for oncocytomas of the minor salivary glands. Recurrence is rare.

ONCOCYTOMA (OXYPHILIC ADENOMA)

The oncocytoma is a benign salivary gland tumor composed of large epithelial cells known as oncocytes. It is a rare neoplasm, representing approximately 1% of all salivary tumors.

Clinical Features

The oncocytoma is predominantly a tumor of older adults, with peak prevalence in the eighth decade of life. A slight female predilection has been observed but may not be significant. Oncocytomas occur primarily in the major salivary glands, especially the parotid gland, which accounts for about 85% to 90% of all cases. Oncocytomas of the minor salivary glands are exceedingly rare. The tumor appears as a firm, slowly growing, painless mass that rarely exceeds 4 cm in diameter. Parotid oncocytomas usually are found in the superficial lobe and are clinically indistinguishable from other benign tumors. On occasion, bilateral tumors can occur, although these may represent examples of multinodular oncocytic hyperplasia (oncocytosis).

Histopathologic Features

The oncocytoma is usually a well-circumscribed tumor that is composed of sheets of large polyhedral cells (oncocytes), with abundant granular, eosinuphilic cytoplasm. Sometimes these cells form an alveolar or glandular pattern. The cells have centrally located nuclei that can vary from small and hyper chromatic to large and vesicular. Little stroma is present, usually in the form of thin fibrovascular septa. An associated lymphocytic infiltrate may be noted. The granularity of the cells is created by an overabundance of mitochondria, which can be demonstrated by electron microscopy. These granules also can be identified on light microscopic examination with a phospho-tungstic acid-hematoxylin (PTAH) stain. The cells also contain glycogen, as evidenced by their positive staining with the periodic acid-Schiff (PAS) technique but by negative PAS staining after digestion with diastase.

Oncocytomas may contain variable numbers of cells with a clear cytoplasm. In rare instances, these clear cells may compose most of the lesion and create difficulty in distinguishing the tumor from other clear cell salivary gland tumors that have a low-grade malignant potential.

Treatment and Prognosis

Oncocytomas are best treated by surgical excision. In the parotid gland, this usually entails partial parotidectomy (lobectomy) to avoid violation of the tumor capsule. The facial nerve should be preserved whenever possible. For tumors in the submandibular gland, treatment consists of total removal of the gland. Oncocytomas of the oral minor salivary glands should be removed with a small margin of normal surrounding tissue. The prognosis after removal is good, with a low rate of recurrence. However, oncocytomas of the sinonasal glands can be locally aggressive and have been considered to be low-grade malignancies. Rare examples of histopathologically malignant oncocytomas (oncocytic carcinoma) also have been reported. These carcinomas have a relatively poor prognosis.

ONCOCYTOSIS (NODULAR ONCOCYTIC HYPERPLASIA)

Oncocytic metaplasia is the transformation of ductal and acinar cells to oncocytes. Such cells are uncommon before the age of 50; however, as people get older, occasional oncocytes are common findings in the salivary glands. Focal oncocytic metaplasia also may be a feature of other salivary gland tumors. Oncocytosis refers to both the proliferation and accumulation of oncocytes within salivary gland tissue. It may mimic a tumor, both clinically and microscopically, but it also is considered to be a metaplastic process rather than a neoplastic one.

Clinical Features

Oncocytosis is found primarily in the parotid gland; however, in rare instances, it may involve the submandibular or minor salivary glands. It can be an incidental finding in otherwise normal salivary gland tissue, but it may be extensive enough to produce clinical swelling. Usually the proliferation is multifocal and nodular, but sometimes the entire gland can be replaced by oncocytes. As with other oncocytic proliferations, oncocytosis occurs most frequently in older adults.

Histopathologic Features

Microscopic examination usually reveals focal nodular collections of oncocytes within the salivary gland tissue. These enlarged cells are polyhedral and demonstrate abundant granular, eosinophilic cytoplasm as a result of the proliferation of mitochondria. On occasion, these cells may have a clear cytoplasm from the accumulation of glycogen. The multifocal nature of the proliferation may be confused with that of a metastatic tumor, especially when the oncocytes are clear in appearance.

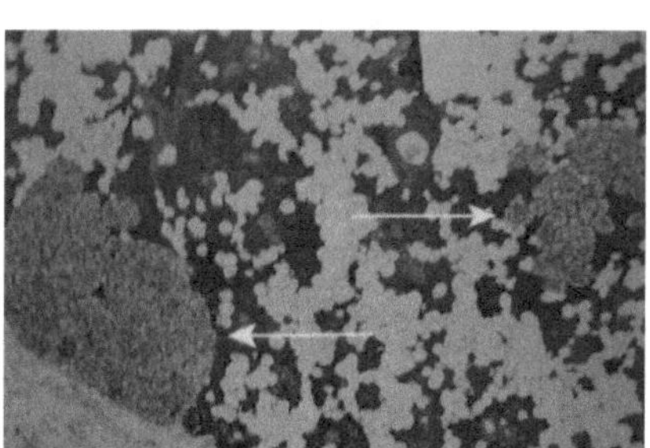

Treatment and Prognosis

Oncocytosis is a benign condition and often is discovered only as an incidental finding. No further treatment is necessary, and the prognosis is excellent.

WARTHIN TUMOR (PAPILLARY CYSTADENOMA LYMPHOMATOSUM)

Warthin tumor is a benign neoplasm that occurs almost exclusively in the parotid gland. Although it is much less common than the pleomorphic adenoma, it represents the second most common benign parotid tumor, accounting for 5% to 14% of all parotid neoplasms. The name adenolymphoma also has been used for this tumor; but this term should be avoided because it overemphasizes the lymphoid component and may give the mistaken impression that the lesion is a type of lymphoma. The pathogenesis of these tumors is uncertain. The traditional hypothesis suggests that they arise from heterotrophic salivary gland tissue found within parotid lymph nodes. However, it also has been suggested that these tumors may develop from a proliferation of salivary gland ductal epithelium that is associated with secondary formation of lymphoid tissue. Several recent papers have supported this latter theory, including studies that have found cytogenetic abnormalities in the epithelial component. A number of studies have demonstrated a strong association between the development of this tumor and smoking. Smokers have an eightfold greater risk for Warthin tumor than do nonsmokers. Epstein-Barr virus also has been implicated in the pathogenesis of Warthin tumor.

Clinical Features

The Warthin tumor usually appears as a slowly growing, painless, nodular mass of the parotid gland. It may be firm or fluctuant to palpation. The tumor most frequently occurs in the tail of the parotid near the angle of the mandible, and it may be noted for many months before the patient seeks a diagnosis. One unique feature is the tendency of Warthin tumor to occur bilaterally, which has been noted in 5% to 14% of cases. Most of these bilateral tumors do not occur simultaneously but are metachronous (occurring at different times).

In rare instances, the Warthin tumor has been reported within the submandibular gland or minor salivary glands. However, because the lymphoid component is often less pronounced in these extra parotid sites, the pathologist should exercise caution to avoid over diagnosis of a lesion better classified as a papillary cystadenoma or salivary duct cyst with oncocytic ductal metaplasia. Warthin tumor most often occurs in older adults, with a peak prevalence in the sixth and seventh decades of life. The observed frequency of this tumor is much lower in blacks than in whites. Most studies show a decided male predilection, with some early studies demonstrating a male-to-female ratio up to 10 to I. However, more recent investigations show a more balanced sex ratio. Because Warthin tumors have been associated with cigarette smoking, this changing sex ratio may be a reflection of the increased prevalence of smoking in females over the past few decades. This association with smoking also may help explain the frequent bilaterality of the tumor, because any tumorigenic effects of smoking might be manifested in both parotids.

Histopathologic Features

The Warthin tumor has one of the most distinctive histopathologic patterns of any tumor in the body. Although the term papillary cystadenoma lymphomatosum is cumbersome, it accurately describes the salient microscopic features.

The tumor is composed of a mixture of ductal epithelium and a lymphoid stroma. The epithelium is oncocytic in nature, forming uniform rows of cells surrounding cystic spaces. The cells have abundant, finely granular eosinophilic cytoplasm and are arranged in two layers. The inner luminal layer consists of tall columnar cells with centrally placed, palisaded, and slightly hyperchromatic nuclei. Beneath this is a second layer of cuboidal or polygonal cells with more vesicular nuclei. The lining epithelium demonstrates multiple papillary infoldings that protrude into the cystic spaces. Focal areas of squamous metaplasia or mucous cell prosoplasia may be seen. The epithelium is supported by a lymphoid stroma that frequently shows germinal center formation.

Treatment and Prognosis

Surgical removal is the treatment of choice for patients with Warthin tumor. The procedure usually is easily accomplished because of the superficial location of the tumor. Some surgeons prefer local resection with minimal surrounding tissue; others opt for superficial parotidectomy to avoid violating the tumor capsule and because a tentative diagnosis may not be known preoperatively. A 6% to 12% recurrence rate has been reported. Many authors, however, believe that the tumor is frequently multicentric in nature; therefore, it is difficult to determine whether these are true recurrences or secondary tumor sites. Malignant Warthin tumors (carcinoma ex papillary cystadenoma lymphomatosum) have been reported but are exceedingly rare.

DUCTALPAPILLOMAS (SIALADENOMA PAPILLIFERUM; INTRADUCTAL PAPILLOMA; INVERTED DUCTAL PAPILLOMA)

A number of salivary gland tumors can be characterized microscopically by a papillomatous pattern, the most common being Warthin tumor (papillary cystadenoma lymphomatosum). The sialadenoma papilliferum, intraductal papilloma, and inverted ductal papilloma are three rare salivary tumors that also show unique papillomatous features. It also should be mentioned that, on occasion, the common squamous papilloma of the oral mucosa will arise at the site where a minor salivary gland duct merges with the surface epithelium. Because of this location, such squamous papillomas also contain scattered mucous cells within the exophytic papillary growth, and these lesions have sometimes been called "ductal papillomas". However, it should be emphasized that these lesions are viral (human papiliomavirus [HPV]) surface papillomas and not primary salivary gland tumors,

Clinical Features

The sialadenoma papilliferum most commonly arises from the minor salivary glands, especially on the palate, although it also has been reported in the parotid gland. It usually is seen in older adults and has a 1.5:1 male-to-female ratio. The tumor appears as an exophytic, papillary surface growth that is clinically similar to the common squamous papilloma.

The intraductal papilloma is an ill-defined lesion that often has been confused with other salivary gland lesions, such as the papillary cystadenoma. It usually occurs in adults and is most common in the minor salivary glands, where it appears as a submucosal swelling.

The inverted ductal papilloma is a rare tumor that has been described only in the minor salivary glands of adults' .The lower lip and mandibular vestibule are the most common locations. The lesion usually appears as an asymptomatic submucosal nodule, which sometimes may show a pit-or indentation in the overlying surface mucosa.

Histopathologic Features

At low power, the sialadenoma papilliferum is somewhat similar to the squamous papilloma, exhibiting multiple exophytic papillary projections that are covered by stratified squamous epithelium. This epithelium is contiguous with a proliferation of papillomatous ductal epithelium found below the surface and extending downward into the deeper connective tissues. Multiple ductal lumina are formed, which characteristically are lined by a double-rowed layer of cells consisting of a luminal layer of tall columnar cells and a basilar layer of smaller cuboidal cells. These ductal cells often have an oncocytic appearance. An inflammatory infiltrate of plasma cells, lymphocytes, and neutrophils is characteristically present. Because of their microscopic similarity, this tumor has been considered to be an analogue of the cutaneous syringocystadenoma papilliferum. The intraductal papilloma exhibits a dilated, unicystic structure that is located below the mucosal surface. It is lined by a single or double row of cuboidal or columnar epithelium, which has multiple arborizing papillary projections into the cystic lumen. In contrast, the inverted ductal papilloma is composed primarily of a proliferation of squamoid epithelium with multiple thick, bulbous papillary projections that fill the ductal lumen.

This epithelium may be contiguous with the overlying mucosal epithelium, communicating with the surface through a small pore like opening. Although the tumor is primarily squamous in nature, the luminal lining cells of the papillary projections are often cuboidal or columnar in shape, with scattered mucus-producing cells.

Treatment and Prognosis

All three forms of ductal papilloma are best treated by conservative surgical excision. Recurrence is rare.

SEBACEOUS ADENOMA

Sebaceous adenomas are rare. These lesions are derived from sebaceous glands located within salivary gland tissue. The parotid gland is the most commonly involved gland.

Pathology

Cells derived from sebaceous glands are present. Benign forms contain well-differentiated sebaceous cells whereas malignant forms consist of more poorly differentiated cells.

Treatment

Removal of the involved gland is the treatment of choice. Intraoral lesions are surgically removed with a border of normal tissue.

MALIGNANT NEOPLASMS

There are several ways to classify' salivary gland malignancies.

1. According to relative frequency, and
2. According to biologic behavior

Malignant tumors

MUCOEPIDERMOID CARCINOMA

The mucoepidermoid carcinoma is one of the most common salivary gland malignancies. Because of its highly variable biologic potential, it was originally called mucoepidermoid tumor. The term recognized one subset that acted in a malignant fashion and a second group that appeared to behave in a benign fashion with favorable prognosis. However, it was later recognized that even low-grade tumors occasionally could exhibit malignant behavior; therefore, the term mucoepidermoid carcinoma is the preferred designation.

Clinical Features

Most studies show that the mucoepidermoid carcinoma is the most common malignant salivary gland neoplasm. In the United States, it makes up 10% of all major gland tumors and 15% to 21 % of minor gland tumors. However, British studies have shown a much lower relative frequency, with mucoepidermoid carcinoma accounting for only I % to 2% of major gland neoplasms and 9% of minor gland tumors. Perhaps a true geographic difference exists in the prevalence of this lesion.

The tumor occurs fairly evenly over a wide age range, extending from the second to seventh decades of life. Rarely is it seen in the first decade of life. However, mucoepidermoid carcinoma is the most common malignant salivary gland tumor in children. A slight female predilection has been noted. Some tumors have been associated with a previous history of radiation therapy to the head and neck region.

The mucoepidermoid carcinoma is most common in the parotid gland and usually appears as an asymptomatic swelling. Most patients are aware of the lesion for a year or less, although some report a mass of many years' duration. Pain or facial nerve palsy may develop, usually in association with high-grade tumors. The minor glands constitute the second most common site, especially the palate. Minor gland tumors also typically appear as asymptomatic swellings, which are sometimes fluctuant and have a blue or red color that can be mistaken clinically for a mucocele. Although the lower lip, floor of mouth, tongue, and retromolar pad areas are uncommon locations for salivary gland neoplasia, the mucoepidermoid carcinoma is the most common salivary tumor in each of these sites. Intraosseous tumors also may develop in the jaws.

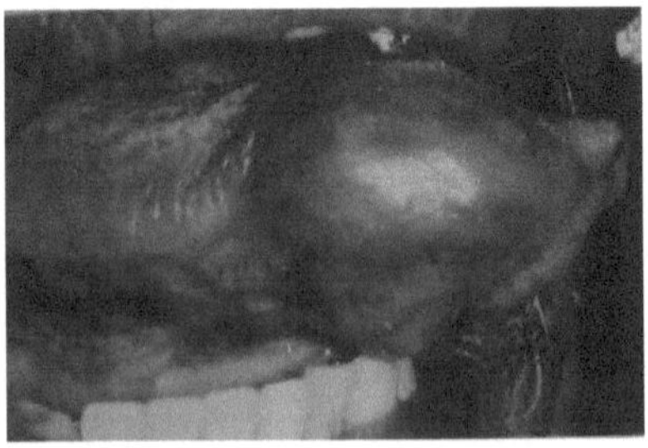

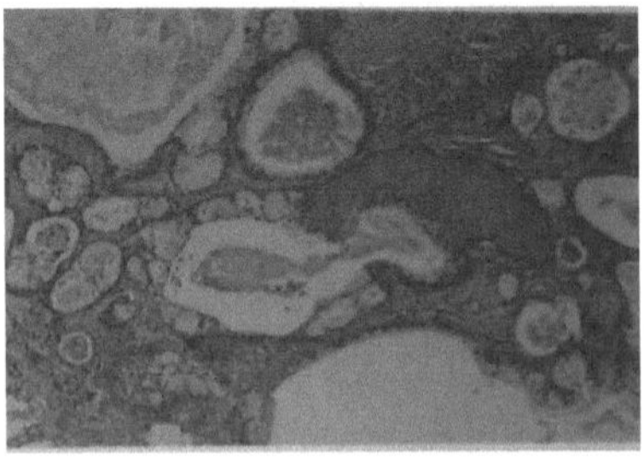

Histopathologic Features

As its name implies, the mucoepidermoid carcinoma is composed of a mixture of mucus-producing cells and squamous (epidermoid) cells, the mucous cells vary in shape but contain abundant foamy cytoplasm that stains positively with mucin stains, The epidermoid cells are characterized by squamoid features, often demonstrating a polygonal shape, intercellular bridges, and, rarely, keratinization. In additions third type of cell is typically present—the intermediate cell. This cell is basaloid in appearance and is believed to be a progenitor of the mucous and epidermoid cells. Some tumors also show variable numbers of clear cells, which sometimes can predominate the microscopic picture. An associated lymphoid infiltrate is not unusual and may be so prominent in some cases that the lesion can be mistaken for a metastatic tumor within a lymph node.

Traditionally, mucoepidermoid carcinomas have been categorized into one of three histopathologic grades based on the following:

1. Amount of cyst formation
2. Degree of cytologic atypia
3. Relative numbers of mucous, epidermoid, and intermediate cells

Low-grade tumors show prominent cyst formation, minimal cellular atypia, and a relatively high proportion of mucous cells. High-grade tumors consist of solid islands of squamous and intermediate cells, which can demonstrate considerable pleomorphism and mitotic activity. Mucus-producing cells may be infrequent, and [he tumor sometimes can be difficult to distinguish from squamous cell carcinoma.

Intermediate-grade tumors show features that fall between those of the low-grade and high-grade neoplasms. Cyst formation occurs but is less prominent than that observed in low-grade tumors. All three major cell types arc present, but the intermediate cells usually predominate. Cellular atypia may or may not be observed.

However, some experts have found that the relative proportion of the three different cell types does not correlate with prognosis. Instead, they have identified five significant microscopic parameters, to which relative point values have been assigned to determine the grade of the tumor.

Mucoepidermoid Carcinoma: Grading Parameters and Point Values

PARAMETER	POINT VALUE
Intracystic component <20%	+2
Neural invasion present	+2
Necrosis present	+3
Four or more mitoses per 10	+3
HPF Anaplasia present	+4

GRADE	TOTAL POINT SCORE
Low	0-4
Intermediate	5-6
High	7-14

Treatment and Prognosis

The treatment of mucoepidermoid carcinoma is predicated by the location, histopathologic grade, and clinical stage of the tumor. Early-stage tumors of the parotid often can be treated by subtotal parotidectomy with preservation of the facial nerve. Advanced tumors may necessitate total removal of the parotid gland, with sacrifice of the facial nerve. Submandibular gland tumors are treated by total removal of the gland. Mucoepidermoid carcinomas of the minor glands usually are treated by assured surgical excision. For low-grade neoplasms, only a modest margin of surrounding normal tissue may need to be removed, but high-grade or large tumors warrant wider resection, similar to that required for squamous cell carcinomas. If there is underlying bone destruction, the involved bone must be excised.

Radical neck dissection is indicated for patients with clinical evidence of metastatic disease and also may be considered for patients with larger or high-grade tumors. Postoperative radiation therapy also may be used for more aggressive tumors.

The prognosis depends on the grade and stage of the tumor. Patients with low-grade tumors generally have a good prognosis. For most primary sites, local recurrences or regional metastases are uncommon, and around 90% to 95% of patients are cured. The prognosis for those with intermediate-grade tumors is slightly worse than that for low-grade tumors. The outlook for patients with high-grade tumors is guarded, with only 30% to 54% of patients surviving.

For unknown reasons, submandibular gland tumors are associated with a poorer outlook than those in the parotid gland. Mucoepidermoid carcinomas of the oral minor salivary glands generally have a good prognosis, probably because they are mostly low- to intermediate-grade tumors. However, tumors of the tongue and floor of the mouth are less predictable and may exhibit more aggressive behavior.

INTRAOSSEOUS MUCOEPIDERMOID CARCINOMA (CENTRAL MUCOEPIDERMOID CARCINOMA)

On rare occasions, salivary gland tumors arise centrally within the jaws. The most common and best-recognized intrabony salivary tumor is the intraosseous mucoepidermoid carcinoma. However, other salivary tumors have been reported to develop within the jaws, including adenoid cystic carcinoma, benign and malignant mixed tumors, adenocarcinoma, acinic cell adenocarcinoma, and monomorphic adenoma.

Several hypotheses have been proposed to explain the pathogenesis of intraosseous salivary tumors. One theory suggests that they may arise from ectopic salivary gland tissue that was developmentally entrapped within the jaws. However, the discovery of ectopic salivary tissue is uncommon in biopsy specimens from the jaws and, therefore, this seems an unlikely source for most intrabony salivary tumors. Some maxillary tumors may arise from glands of the sinus lining, but this is often difficult to prove or disprove. The most likely source for most intraosseous tumors is odontogenic epithelium. Mucus-producing cells are common in odontogenic cyst linings, especially dentigerous cysts. In addition, many intraosseous mucoepidermoid carcinomas develop in association with impacted teeth or odontogenic cysts.

Clinical and Radiographic Features

Intraosseous mucoepidermoid carcinomas are most common in middle-aged adults and demonstrate a slight female predilection. They are three times more common in the mandible than in the maxilla and are most often seen in the molar-ramus area. The most frequent presenting symptom is cortical swelling, although some lesions may be discovered as incidental findings on radiographs. Pain, trismus, and paresthesia are reported less frequently.

Radiographs usually reveal either unilocular or multilocular radiolucency with well-defined borders. However, some examples are characterized by a more irregular and ill-defined area of bone destruction, some cases is associated with an unerupted tooth and, therefore, clinically may suggest an odontogenic cyst or tumor.

Histopathologic Features

The microscopic appearance of intraosseous mucoepidermoid carcinoma is similar to that of its soft tissue counterpart. Most tumors are low-grade lesions, although high-grade mucoepidermoid carcinomas also have been reported within the jaws.

Treatment and Prognosis

The primary treatment modality for patients with intraosseous mucoepidermoid carcinoma is surgery; adjunctive radiation therapy also sometimes is used. Radical surgical resection offers a better chance for cure than do more conservative procedures, such as enucleation or curettage. The local recurrence rate with conservative treatment is 40%, in contrast to I 3% for more radical treatment. Metastasis has been reported in about 12% of cases.

The overall prognosis is fairly good; around 10% of patients die, usually as a result of local recurrence of the tumor.

ACINIC CELL ADENOCARCINOMA

The acinic cell adenocarcinoma is a salivary gland malignancy with cells that show serous acinar differentiation. Because many of these tumors act in a non-aggressive fashion and are associated with a good prognosis, this neoplasm formerly was called acinic cell tumor, a nonspecific designation that did not indicate whether the lesion was benign or malignant. However, because some of these tumors do metastasize or recur and cause death, it is generally agreed today that acinic cell adenocarcinoma should be considered a low-grade malignancy.

Clinical Features

Around 85% of all acinic cell adenocarcinomas occur in the parotid gland, a logical finding because this is the largest gland and one that is composed entirely of serous elements. Most surveys have shown that this neoplasm makes up 1 % to 3% of all parotid tumors, although one study showed it represented 8.6% of all parotid tumors. It is much less common in the sub-mandibular gland, which is the site for only 2.7% to 4% of these tumors. About 9% of all acinic cell adenocarcinomas develop in the oral minor salivary glands, with the buccal mucosa, lips, and palate being the most common sites , overall, around 2% to 6.5% of all minor salivary gland tumors are acinic cell adenocarcinomas.

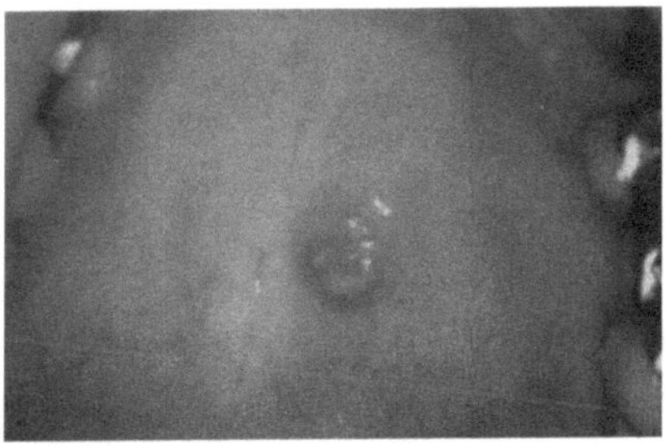 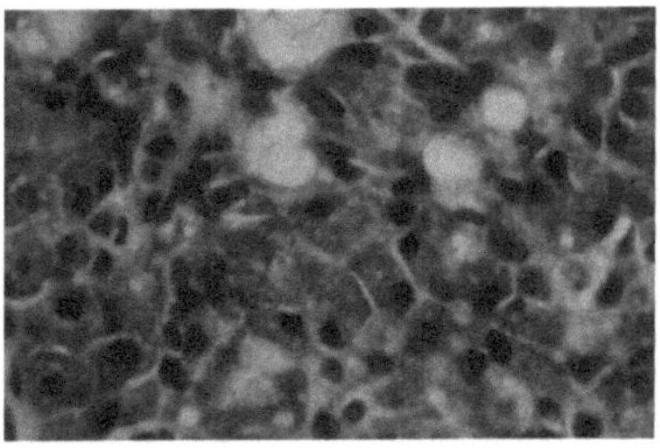

The tumor occurs over a broad age range, with a relatively even peak prevalence stretching from the second to the seventh decades of life; the mean age is in the middle 40s. Approximately 60% of cases occur in women. The tumor usually appears as a slowly growing mass, and the lesion often is appears for many months or years before a diagnosis is made. The tumor may be otherwise asymptomatic, although associated pain or tenderness sometimes is reported. Facial nerve paralysis is an infrequent but ominous sign for parotid tumors.

Histopathologic Features

Acinic cell adenocarcinomas are highly variable in their microscopic appearance. The tumor often is well circumscribed and sometimes may even appear encapsulated; however, some tumors exhibit an infiltrative growth pattern. The most characteristic cell is one with features of the serous acinar cell, with abundant granular basophilic cytoplasm and a round, darkly stained eccentric nucleus. These cells arc fairly uniform in appearance and mitotic activity is uncommon. Other cells may resemble intercalated duct cells, and some tumors also have cells with a clear, vacuolated cytoplasm.

Several growth patterns may be seen. The solid variety consists of numerous well-differentiated acinar cells arranged in a pattern that resembles normal parotid gland tissue. In the micro cystic variety, multiple small cystic spaces are created that may contain some mucinous or eosinophilic material. In the papillary-cystic variety, larger cystic areas are formed that are lined by epithelium having papillary projections into the cystic spaces. The follicular variety has an appearance similar to that of thyroid tissue. A lymphoid infiltrate is not unusual, sometimes with germinal center formation.

Treatment and Prognosis

Acinic cell adenocarcinomas confined to the superficial lobe of the parotid gland are best treated by lobectomy; for those in the deep lobe, total parotidectomy is usually necessary.

The facial nerve may need to be sacrificed if it is involved by tumor. Submandibular tumors are managed by total removal of the gland, and minor gland tumors are treated with assured surgical excision. Lymph node dissection is not indicated unless there is clinical evidence of metastatic disease. Adjunctive radiation therapy may be considered for uncontrolled local disease. The acinic cell adenocarcinoma is associated with one of the better prognoses of any of the malignant salivary g\and tumors. Approximately one third of patients have recurrences locally, and metastases develop in 10% to 15% of patients. From 6% to 26% of patients die of their disease. The prognosis for minor gland tumors is better than that for tumors arising in the major glands.

MALIGNANT MIXED TUMORS (CARCINOMA EX PLEOMORPHIC ADENOMA; CARCINOMA EX MIXED TUMOR; CARCINOSARCOMA; METASTASIZINC MIXED TUMOR)

Malignant mixed tumors represent malignant counterparts to the benign mixed tumor or pleomorphic adenoma. These uncommon neoplasms constitute 2% to 6% of all salivary tumors and can be divided into three categories:

1. Carcinoma ex pleomorphic adenoma (carcinoma ex mixed tumor)
2. Carcinosarcoma
3. Metastasizing mixed tumor

The most common of these is the carcinoma ex pleomorphic adenoma, which is characterized by malignant transformation of the epithelial component of a previously benign pleomorphic adenoma. The carcinosarcoma is a rare "mixed" tumor in which both carcinomatous and sarcomatous elements are present. The metastasizing mixed tumor has histopathologic features that are identical to the common pleomorphic adenoma (mixed tumor). In spite of its benign appearance, however, the lesion metastasizes. The metastatic tumor also has a benign microscopic appearance, usually similar to that of the primary lesion.

Clinical Features

Carcinoma ex pleomorphic adenoma

There is fairly convincing evidence that the carcinoma ex pleomorphic adenoma represents a malignant transformation within what was previously a benign neoplasm. First of all, the mean age of patients with this tumor is about 15 years older than that for the benign pleomorphic adenoma. It is most common in middle-aged and older adults, with peak prevalence in the sixth to eighth decades of life. In addition, patients may report that a mass has been present for many years, sometimes undergoing a recent rapid growth with associated pain or ulceration. However, some tumors may have a short duration. The histopathologic features, which are discussed later, also support malignant transformation of a benign pleomorphic adenoma. It has been noted that the risk for malignant change in a pleomorphic adenoma increases with the duration of the tumor.

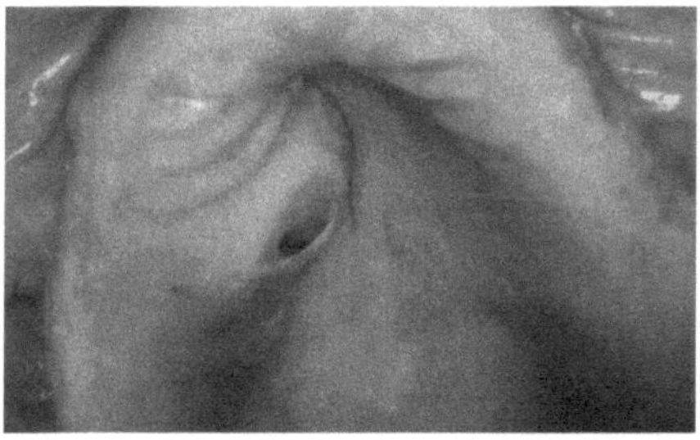

Over 80% of cases of carcinoma ex pleomorphic adenoma are seen within the major glands, primarily the parotid gland. Nearly two thirds of minor salivary gland cases occur on the palate. There is a slight female predilection. Although pain or recent rapid growth is not unusual, many cases present as a painless mass that is indistinguishable from a benign tumor. Parotid tumors may produce facial nerve palsy.

Carcinosarcoma

The carcinosarcoma is an extremely rare tumor. Most cases have been reported in the parotid gland, but the lesion also has been seen in the sub-mandibular gland and minor salivary glands. The clinical signs and symptoms are similar to those of the carcinoma ex pleomorphic adenoma. Some patients have a previous history of a benign pleomorphic adenoma, although other cases appear to arise de novo.

Metastasizing mixed tumor

The metastasizing mixed tumor is also quite rare. As with other malignant mixed tumors, most cases originate in the parotid gland, but the primary tumor also may occur in the submandibular gland or minor salivary glands. Metastases have been found most frequently in the bones or lung, but they also can occur in other sites, such as regional lymph nodes or the liver. Most patients have a history of a benign mixed tumor, which may have been excised many years earlier. Many times the primary tumor exhibits multiple recurrences before metastasis occurs.

Histopathologic Features

Carcinoma ex pleomorphic adenoma

The carcinoma ex pleomorphic adenoma shows a variable microscopic appearance. Areas of typical benign pleomorphic adenoma usually can be found and may constitute most or only a small portion of the lesion. Within the tumor are areas of malignant degeneration of the epithelial component, characterized by cellular pleomorphism and abnormal mitotic activity. This change is most often in the form of a poorly differentiated adeno-carcinoma, but other patterns also can develop, including polymorphous low-grade adenocarcinoma, mucoepidermoid carcinoma, and adenoid cystic carcinoma. The malignant component often has an aggressive growth pattern, with capsular invasion and infiltration into surrounding tissues. However, in rare instances it is discovered as a small focus within the center of an encapsulated mixed tumor. Because such tumors have a markedly better prognosis than invasive tumors, they have been designated as noninvasive pleomorphic adenoma..

Carcinosarcoma

The carcinosarcoma is a biphasic tumor, demonstrating both carcinomatous and sarcomatous areas. The epithelial component usually consists of a poorly differentiated adenocarcinoma or an undifferentiated carcinoma. The sarcomatous portion often predominates the tumor and is usually in the form of chondrosarcoma but also may show characteristics of osteosarcoma, fibrosarcoma, liposarcoma, or malignant fibrous histiocytoma. Some lesions have evidence of an origin from a benign mixed tumor.

Metastasized mixed tumor

The metastasizing mixed tumor has microscopic features of a benign pleomorphic adenoma, within both the primary and metastatic sites. Malignant histopathologic changes are not observed.

Treatment and Prognosis

Carcinoma ex pleomorphic adenoma

Invasive carcinoma ex pleomorphic adenoma usually is best treated by wide excision, possibly in conjunction with local lymph node dissection and adjunctive radiation therapy. The prognosis is guarded; the overall 5-year survival rate ranges from 25% to 65%, but this rate drops to 10% to 35% at 15 years. The prognosis is related to the histopathologic subtype of the malignant component. One study showed that well-differentiated carcinomas, such as polymorphous low-grade adenocarcinoma, have nearly a 90% 5-year survival rate. In contrast, the outlook is much worse for patients with tumors that are poorly differentiated or that have invaded more than 8 mm beyond the residual capsule or benign residual tumor. However, for cases of in situ (noninvasive) carcinoma ex mixed tumor, the prognosis is similar to that for benign mixed tumor.

Carcinosarcoma

Carcinosarcomas are treated by radical surgical excision, which may be combined with radiation therapy and chemotherapy. The prognosis is poor, with around 75% of patients either dying from their disease or suffering from recurrent local tumor or metastases.

Metastasizing mixed tumor

The treatment for a metastasizing mixed tumor consists of surgical excision of both the primary tumor and metastatic sites. A mortality rate of 22% has been reported.

ADENOID CYSTIC CARCINOMA

The adenoid cystic carcinoma is one of the more common and best-recognized salivary malignancies. Because of its distinctive histopathologic features, it was originally called a cylindroma, and this term still is used sometimes as a synonym for this neoplasm. However, use of the term cylindroma probably should be avoided today because the same term is used for a skin adnexal tumor that has a markedly different clinical presentation and prognosis,

Clinical and Radiographic features

The adenoid cystic carcinoma can occur in any salivary gland site, but approximately 50% develop within the minor salivary glands. The palate is the most common site for minor gland tumors. The remaining tumors are found mostly in the parotid and submandibular glands, with a fairly even distribution between these two sites. On an individual basis, however, a striking difference can be seen among the various glands. In the parotid gland, the adenoid cystic carcinoma is relatively rare, constituting only 2% to 3% of all tumors. In the submandibular gland, this tumor accounts for 12% to 17% of all tumors and is the most common malignancy. It is also relatively common among palatal salivary neoplasms; it represents 8% to 15% of all such tumors. The lesion is most common in middle-aged adults and is rare in people younger than age 20. There is a fairly equal sex distribution, although some studies have shown a slight female predilection.

The adenoid cystic carcinoma usually appears as a slowly growing mass. Pain is a common and important finding, occasionally occurring early in the course of the disease before there is a noticeable swelling. Patients often complain of a constant, low-grade, dull ache, which gradually increases in intensity. Facial nerve paralysis may develop with parotid tumors. Palatal tumors can be smooth surfaced or ulcerated. Tumors arising in the palate or maxillary sinus may show radiographic evidence of bone destruction.

Histopathologic Features

The adenoid cystic carcinoma is composed of a mixture of myoepithelial cells and ductal cells that can have a varied arrangement. Three major patterns are recognized:

(I) Cribriform,

(2) Tubular, and

(3) Solid.

Usually a combination of these is seen, and the tumor is classified based on the predominant pattern.

The cribriform pattern is the most classic and best-recognized appearance, characterized by islands of hasaloid epithelial cells that contain multiple cylindric, cystlike spaces resembling Swiss cheese. These spaces often contain a mildly basophilic mucoid material, a hyalinized eosinophilic product, or a combined mucoid-hyalinized appearance. Sometimes the hyalinized material also surrounds these cribriform islands, or small strands of tumor are found embedded within this hyalinized "stroma." The tumor cells are small and cuboidal, exhibiting deeply basophilic nuclei and little cytoplasm. These cells are fairly uniform in appearance, and mitotic activity is rarely seen.

In the tubular pattern, the tumor cells are similar but occur as multiple small ducts or tubules within a hyalinized stroma. The tubular lumina can be lined by one to several layers of cells, and sometimes both a layer of ductal cells and myoepithelial cells can be discerned.

The solid variant consists of larger islands or sheets of tumor cells that demonstrate little tendency toward duct or cyst formation. Unlike the cribriform and tubular patterns, cellular pleomorphism and mitotic activity, as well as focal necrosis in the center of the tumor islands, may be observed.

A highly characteristic feature of adenoid cystic carcinoma is its tendency to show perineural invasion, which probably corresponds to the common clinical finding of pain in these patients. Sometimes the cells appear to have a swirling arrangement around nerve bundles. However, perineural invasion is not pathognomonic for adenoid cystic carcinoma; it also may be seen in other salivary malignancies, especially polymorphous low-grade adenocarcinomas.

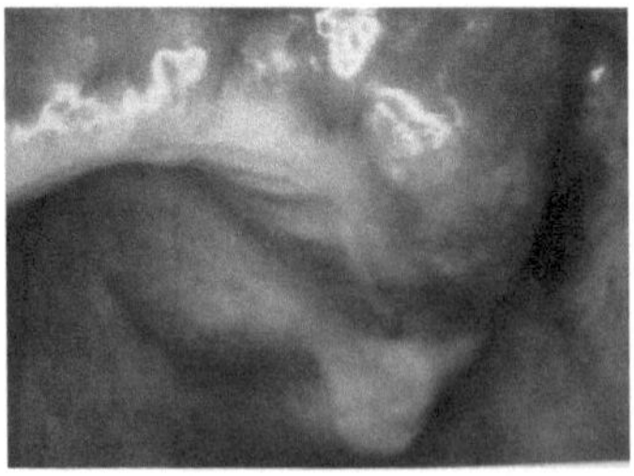

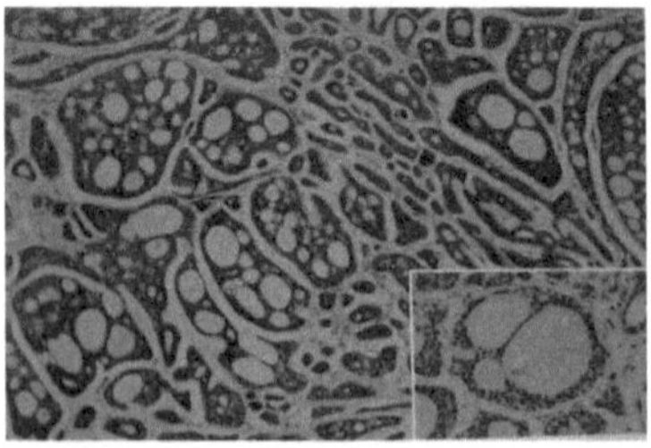

Treatment and Prognosis

Adenoid cystic carcinoma is a relentless tumor that is prone to local recurrence and eventual distant metastasis. Surgical excision is usually the treatment of choice, and adjunct radiation therapy may slightly improve patient survival in some cases. Because metastasis to regional lymph nodes is uncommon, radical neck dissection typically is not indicated. Because of the poor overall prognosis, regardless of treatment, clinicians should be cautioned against needlessly aggressive and mutilating surgical procedures for large tumors or cases already showing metastases.

Because the tumor is prone to late recurrence and metastasis, the 5-year survival rate has little significance and docs not equate to a cure. The 5-year survival rate may be as high as 70%, but this rate continues to decrease over time. By 20 years, only 20% of patients are still alive. Tumors with a solid histopathologic pattern are associated with a worse outlook than those with a cribriform or tubular arrangement. With respect to site, the prognosis is poorest for tumors arising in the maxillary sinus and submandibular gland. Most studies have shown that microscopic identification of perineural invasion has little effect on the prognosis. Death usually results from local recurrence or distant metastases. Tumors of the palate or maxillary sinus eventually may invade upward to the base of the brain. Metastatic spread most commonly occurs to the lungs and bones.

POLYMORPHOUS LOW-GRADE ADENOCARC1NOMA (LOBULAR CARCINOMA; TERMINAL DUCT CARCINOMA)

The polymorphous low-grade adenocarcinoma is a recently recognized type of salivary malignancy that was first described in I983. Before its identification as a distinct entity, examples of this tumor were categorized as pleomorphic adenoma, an unspecified form of adeno-carcinoma, or sometimes adenoid cystic carcinoma. Once recognized as a specific entity, however, it was realized that this tumor possesses distinct clinicopathologic features and is one of the more common minor salivary gland malignancies.

Clinical Features

The polymorphous low-grade adenocarcinoma is almost exclusively a tumor of the minor salivary glands. However, rare examples also have been reported in the major glands, either arising de novo or as the malignant component of a carcinoma ex pleomorphic adenoma. Sixty-five percent occur on the hard or soft palate, with the upper lip and buccal mucosa being the next most common locations. It is most common in older adults, having peak prevalence in two to eighth decades of life. Two thirds of all cases 'occur in females.

The tumor most often appears as a painless mass may have been present for a long time with slow growth. Occasionally, it is associated with bleeding or discomfort. Tumor can erode or infiltrate the underlying bone.

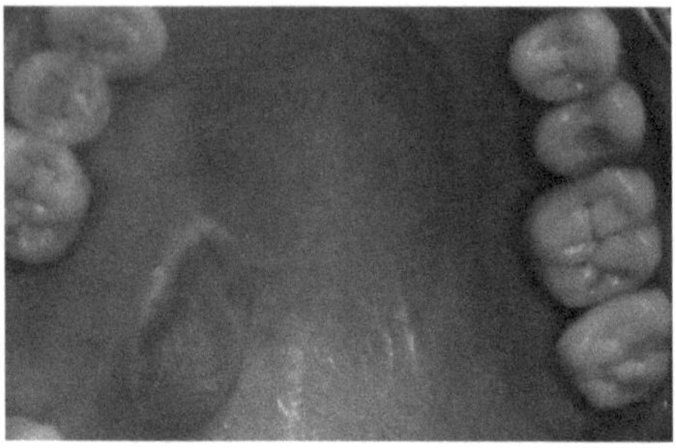

Histopathologic Features

The tumor cells of polymorphous low-grade adenocarcinomas have a deceptively uniform appearance. They are round to polygonal in shape, with indistinct cell borders and pale to eosinophilic cytoplasm. The nuclei may be round, ovoid, or spindled; these nuclei usually arc pale staining, although they can be more basophilic in some areas. The cells can exhibit different growth patterns, nonce, the polymorphous term. The cells may grow in a solid pattern or form cords, ducts, or larger cystic spaces. In some tumors, a cribriform pattern can be produced that mimics adenoid cystic carcinoma. Mitotic figures are uncommon. At low power, the tumor sometimes appears well circumscribed. However, the peripheral cells are usually infiltrative, invading the adjacent tissue in a single-file fashion. Extension into underlying bone or skeletal muscle may be observed. The stroma is often mucoid in nature, or it may demonstrate hyalinization. Perineural invasion is common—another feature that may cause the tumor to be mistaken for adenoid cystic carcinoma. However, a distinction between these two tumors is important because of their vastly different prognoses.

Treatment and Prognosis

The polymorphous low-grade adenocarcinoma is best treated by wide surgical excision, sometimes including resection of the underlying bone. Metastasis to regional lymph nodes is relatively uncommon, occurring in just under 10% of patients. Therefore, radical neck dissection seems unwarranted unless there is clinical evidence of cervical metastases. Distant metastasis is rare.

The overall prognosis is relatively good. Recurrent disease has been reported in 9% to I 7% of all patients, but this usually can be controlled with reexcision. Death from tumor is rare but may occur secondary to direct extension into vital structures. Microscopic identification of perineural invasion does not appear to affect the prognosis.

SALIVARY ADENOCARCINOMA, NOT OTHERWISE SPECIFIED

In spite of the wide variety of salivary gland malignancies that have been specifically identified and categorized, some tumors still defy the existing classification schemes. These tumors usually are designated as salivary adenocarcinomas, not otherwise specified (NOS).

Clinical and Histopathologic Features

Because these adenocarcinomas represent such a diverse group of neoplasms, it is difficult to generalize about their clinical and microscopic features. Like most salivary tumors, they appear to be most common in the parotid gland, followed by the minor glands and the sub-mandibular gland. They may present as asymptomatic masses or cause pain or facial nerve paralysis. The microscopic appearance is highly variable but demonstrates features of a glandular malignancy with evidence of cellular pleomorphism, an infiltrative growth pattern, or both. These tumors exhibit a wide spectrum of differentiation, ranging from well-differentiated, low-grade neoplasms to poorly differentiated, high-grade malignancies. As these tumors are studied more, it should be possible to classify some of them into separate, specific categories and allow more definitive analyses of their clinical and microscopic features.

Treatment and Prognosis

The prognosis for salivary adenocarcinoma (NOS) is guarded, but patients with early-stage, well-differentiated tumors appear to have a better outcome. The survival rate is better for tumors of the oral cavity than for those in the major salivary glands.

Clear Cell Carcinoma

There are four salivary gland tumors that, when poorly fixed, may have areas in which tumor cells exhibit clear cytoplasm, apparently as a result of autolysis of cytoplasmic organelles. There are also two clear cell tumors—clear cell carcinoma and epimyoepithelial carcinoma —that exhibit clear cell changes that are due to cytoplasmic accumulation of glycogen and myofilaments, respectively. Clear cell carcinoma, formerly called Hyalinizing Clear Cell Carcinoma, is a low-grade tumor occurring predominantly in minor salivary glands (80% of cases). Most present as submucosal masses in the palate, although other sites may be affected. Microscopically, the neoplasm is composed of uniform bland cells, predominantly with clear cytoplasm. The pattern is typically trabecular, although nests and sheets of cells may be seen. The tumor cells stain positive for glycogen, but negative for mucin, S-100 protein, and muscle-specific actin. Treatment is by excision, and recurrences are very uncommon.

RARE TUMORS

Epimyoepithelial Carcinoma

Epimyoepithelial carcinoma is a clear cell containing malignancy of salivary gland (predominantly the major glands) origin. It is seen in the seventh and eighth decades of life, and there is a two-to-one female predilection.

A lobular growth is composed of two cell types: abundant clear cells with islands of cuboidal, darkly staining cells form a lumen. Glycogen, actins, and S-100 protein are present in these cells, supporting their myoepithelial origin.

Recurrences have most often been associated with lesions greater than 3 cm. The overall recurrence and metastasis rates suggest that this is a malignancy of intermediate grade.

Salivary Duct Carcinoma

Salivary duct carcinoma is a high-grade malignancy of the major salivary glands. It is characterized clinically by a distinctive predominance in the parotid gland (more than 80% of cases); the submandibular gland accounts for the remainder of cases. Nearly 80% of cases have been recorded in men, and the overall peak incidence is in the seventh decade. The lesion arises as a firm, painless mass. A striking microscopic resemblance to ductal carcinomas originating in the breast is noted, with architectural features that include papillary cribriform and solid growth patterns, along with a desmoplastic stroma and comedo necrosis. Nuclear atypia is noted, but few mitoses are seen. Most tumors have infiltrative margins, with neural invasion evident in approximately 50% of cases.

Surgical excision is the treatment of choice. Large series indicate that more than 50% of patients die of their disease within 5 months to 6 years after treatment. Pulmonary and osseous metastases are often noted.

Basal Cell Adenocarcinoma

Basal cell adenocarcinoma, a rare tumor of the major salivary glands, is believed to be the malignant counterpart of basal cell adenoma. It appears microscopically similar to basal cell adenoma, except that it exhibits an infiltrative growth pattern and has the ability to metastasize. These tumors are composed of nests, cords, and solid zones of basaloid cells. Two cytologic types of cells are often seen: small, compact cells and larger, polygonal cells. The former may often be seen surrounding the latter, often in a palisade fashion. The feature that separates this tumor from basal cell adenoma is the finding of small nests of neoplasm in adjacent normal structures. Infiltration of nerve is also seen. Local recurrence and distant metastasis seem to be distinct potentials for basal cell adenocarcinoma. Nonetheless, this tumor is generally regarded as a low-grade malignancy. With adequate surgical treatment, patients should have a favorable outcome.

Squamous Cell Carcinoma

Squamous cell carcinoma arising within the salivary gland tissue of the major salivary glands. The submandibular gland is most commonly involved, followed by the parotid. Obstructive sialadenitis (more common in the submandibular gland) has been thought to be a predisposing condition. Most patients are in the seventh decade of life or beyond.

Squamous cell carcinomas of the parotid and submandibular glands are generally well to moderately well differentiate with no evidence of mucin production. Metastatic squamous cell carcinoma and high-grade mucoepidermoid carcinoma are usually alternative diagnoses.

Local recurrence and regional lymph node metastasis are common events, and distant metastasis is unusual. Surgery is the treatment of choice. As with most other salivary gland malignancies, ultimate survival relates more to the clinical stage than to histologic differentiate

LYMPHOMA

By definition, "primary lymphoma" describes a situation in which a salivary gland is the first clinical manifestation of the disease. Primary lymphoma of the salivary glands probably arises from lymph tissue within the glands. However, primary lymphoma of the salivary glands is rare. The major forms of lymphoma are non-Hodgkin's lymphoma (NHL) and Hodgkin's disease. NHL is less curable and is often disseminated at diagnosis. There is an increased incidence of NHL in patients with autoimmune disease.

The parotid gland is the most commonly involved gland, followed by the submandibular gland.

Clinical Presentation

This lesion commonly presents as painless gland enlargement or adenopathy.

Treatment

Superficial parotidectomy is recommended for isolated asymptomatic parotid gland masses. A staging workup is required to determine treatment. An initial phase of observation is not uncommon for patients with asymptomatic low-grade disease. Appropriate treatment includes radiation therapy, chemotherapy, or a combination of the two, depending on the staging of the lymphoma.

Surgical Treatment

PAROTIDECTOMY

Since most tumors of the parotid gland occur in the tail region, superficial to the facial nerve, surgical treatment most commonly consists of superficial parotidectomy. The facial nerve is identified at surgery in order to avoid damage. If a tumor is very small, it may be excised with an adequate margin of tissue, leaving the remainder of the superficial lobe. Superficial parotidectomy is also the treatment of choice in cases of low grade malignant salivary tumors.

For high-grade malignant salivary tumors, a total parotidectomy is performed. Unless there is intimate involvement of the tumor with the facial nerve, the nerve may be spared. If the tumor does invade the nerve, resection of the nerve is performed, with immediate reconstruction. Biopsies of any suspicious regional lymph nodes are performed; if the results are positive for malignancy, a modified neck dissection is performed immediately. There is no evidence to support prophylactic neck dissection for malignant tumors of the salivary glands. Complications can occur after parotidectomy. Permanent partial or total facial nerve paralysis occurs in less than 3% of patients, and temporary nerve palsies can occur in 10 to 30% of patients. A salivary fistula or sialocele is a relatively common complication after parotid gland surgery. A sialocele occurs when an edge of the parotid gland capsule is cut and the gland continues to leak fluid, leading to a palpable collection. Pressure dressings can be applied, and an antisialagogue such as glycopyrolate can be given if there are no contraindications. In cases of chronic sialoceles, serial aspirations or drain placement may be carried out in an attempt to expedite resolution. Frey's syndrome is a relatively common complication of parotidectomy. This syndrome presents as gustatory sweating.

When regenerating postganglionic secretory parasympathetic fibers from the parotid gland become mixed with the postganglionic sympathetic fibers to the sweat glands, a condition in which a patient will flush or sweat with salivary stimulation results .Minor's starch-iodine test can be used to demonstrate the area of gustatory sweating. Iodine is applied to the patient's face and is allowed to dry. Starch is then lightly applied to the regions of interest. After a sialagogue is administered, the patient will begin to sweat in the areas of involvement. Wetting the starch and iodine, the sweat will turn the involved areas black. This test aids in delineating the distribution of affected area. Frey's syndrome can occur in as many as 30 to 60% of patients who have undergone parotidectomy. The treatment of this disorder consists of the topical application of antiperspirants or anticholinergics. Botulinum toxin injections have been used to treat Frey's syndrome. However, it is recommended that only experienced clinicians attempt this treatment.

SUBMANDIBULAR, SUBLINGUAL, AND MINOR SALIVARYGLAND SURGERY

Tumors of the submandibular and sublingual glands are treated by total removal of the gland. The loss of salivary flow from a single submandibular gland is negligible, and patients tolerate this procedure well. The risks associated with the removal of the submandibular gland include hemorrhage, infection, and injury to the hypoglossal, lingual, or marginal mandibular nerves.

The treatment of tumors of the minor salivary glands depends on the location and extent of disease. Complete excision is usually sufficient for benign tumors. Complications from the treatment of benign lesions are few. In contrast, the treatment of malignant tumors may involve maxillectomy or composite resection.

CONCLUSION:

With the innumerous number of functions of salivary glands and its secretion namely saliva that we have come across, we can arguably call this secretion namely saliva the champion among the factors that are involved in homeostasis of our body. Since dentistry is basically a material science thorough knowledge is important for us to come out with new innovations so that products we use render maximal service to the patient. Evaluation of salivary gland function should therefore be a routine part of any oral examination in order to manage and prevent serious oral and pharyngeal consequences of salivary gland dysfunction.

REFERENCES:

Text book references:

1) William G. Shafer., Maynard K. Hine, Barnet M. Levy. A Text Book of Oral Pathology. 4th edition, W.B. Saunder's Company.
2) Stuart C. White, Michael J. Paroah. "Oral Radiology Principles and Interpretation". 5th Edition. Mosby
3) R.A. Cawson, E.W. Odell, S. Porter. Cawson's Essentials of Oral Pathology and Oral Medicine. 7th edition. Churchill. Livingstone Elsiver science
4) S.N. Bhaskar. Orban's Oral histology and Embryology 11th Edition. Harcourt Asia PTE Ltd. (Mosby).
5) BKB Berkovitz, G.R. Holland, B.J. Moxham, "Oral Anatomy, Histology and Embryology", 3rd Edition. Mosby.
6) A.R. Tencate. Oral Histology, Development, Structure and Function. 5th Edition.
7) Robert L. Pollack, Edward Kravitz. "Nutrition in Oral health and disease". 1st Edition. Lea and Febiger.
8) Paul W. Goaz, Stuart C. White. "Oral Radiology. Principles and Interpretation". 3rd Edition. Mosby.
9) Martin S. Greenberg and Michael Glick. "Burket's Oral Medicine". 10th Edition. Elsevier India.
10) J.R. Garett, J Ekstrom, LC. Anderson. "Glandular mechanism of salivary secretion". Vol. 10 Karger.

Journals and Articles

1. Andersen SW, Machin D (1997). Acupuncture treatment of patients with radiation-induced xerostomia. Oral Oncol 33: 146±147.
2. Arneberg P, Bjertness E, Storhaug K, Glennas A, Bjerkhoel F (1992). Remaining teeth, oral dryness and dental health habits in middle-aged Norwegian rheumatoid arthritis patients. Comm Dent Oral Epidemiol 20: 292±296.
3. Atkinson JC, Baum BJ (2001). Salivary enhancement: current status and future therapies. J Dent Educ 65: 1096±1101.
4. Atkinson JC, Fox PC (1992). Salivary gland dysfunction. Clin Geriatr Med 8: 499±511.

5. Atkinson JC, Wu A (1994). Salivary gland dysfunction: causes, symptoms, treatment. J Am Dent Assoc 125: 409±416.

6. August M, Wang J, Plante D, Wang CC (1996). Complications associated with therapeutic neck radiation. J Oral Maxillo- fac Surg 54: 1409±1415; Discussion 1415±6.

7. Baum BJ (1981). Evaluation of stimulated parotid saliva flow rate in different age groups. J Dent Res 60: 1292±1296.

8. Baum BJ, Ship JA, Wu AJ (1992). Salivary gland function and aging: a model for studying the interaction of aging and systemic disease. CRC Crit Rev Oral Biol Med 4: 53±64.

9. Baum BJ, Dai Y, Hiramatsu Y, Horn VJ, Ambudkar IS (1993). Signaling mechanisms that regulate saliva formation. Crit Rev Oral Biol Medical 4: 379±384.

10. Baum BJ, Wang S, Cukierman E et al (1999). Re-engineering the functions of a terminally di.erentiated epithelial cell in vivo. Ann NY Acad Sci 875: 294±300.

11. Baum BJ, Goldsmith CM, Hoque AT et al (2000). Salivary glands as a model for craniofacial applications of gene transfer. Int J Oral Max Surg 29: 163±166.

12. Bell M, Askari A, Bookman A et al (1999). Sjogren's syndrome: a critical review of clinical management. J Rheum 26: 2051±2061.

13. Bergdahl M, Bergdahl J (2000). Low unstimulated salivary flow and subjective oral dryness: association with medication, anxiety, depression, and stress. J Dent Res 79: 1652± 1658.

14. Chaushu G, Itzkovitz-Chaushu S, Yefenof E, Slavin S, Or R, Garfunkel AA (1995). A longitudinal follow-up of salivary secretion in bone marrow transplant patients. Oral Surg Oral Med Oral Path Oral Radiol Endod 79: 164±169.

15. Chaushu G, Bercovici M, Dori S et al (2000). Salivary flow and its relation with oral symptoms in terminally ill patients. Cancer 88: 984±987.

16. Chavez EM, Taylor GW, Borrell LN, Ship JA (2000). Salivary function and glycemic control in older persons with diabetes. Oral Surg Oral Med Oral Path Oral Radiol Endod 89: 305±311.

17. Chavez EM, Borrell LN, Taylor GW, Ship JA (2001). A longitudinal analysis of salivary ¯ow in control subjects and older adults with type 2 diabetes. Oral Surg Oral Med Oral Path Oral Radiol Endod 91: 166±173.

18. Conley RR, Tamminga CA, Bartko JJ et al (1998). Olanzapine compared with chlorpromazine in treatment-resistant schi- zophrenia. Am J Psychiatr 155: 914±920.

19. Daniels TE, Whitcher JP (1994). Association of patterns of labial salivary gland in¯ammation with keratoconjunctivitis sicca. Analysis of 618 patients with suspected Sjogren's syndrome. Arthritis Rheum 37: 869±877.

20. Davies AN (2000). A comparison of arti®cial saliva and chewing gum in the management of xerostomia in patients with advanced cancer. Palliat Med 14: 197±203.

21. Davies AN, Daniels C, Pugh R, Sharma K (1998). A comparison of arti®cial saliva and pilocarpine in the
22. management of xerostomia in patients with advanced cancer. Palliat Med 12: 105±111.

23. Davies AN, Singer J (1994). A comparison of arti®cial saliva and pilocarpine in radiation-induced xerostomia. J Laryngol Otol 108: 663±665.

24. Dawes C (1975). Circadian rhythms in the ¯ow rate and composition of unstimulated and stimulated human submandibular saliva. J Physiol 244: 535±548.

MIX
Papier | Fördert gute Waldnutzung
FSC® C083411

Kolibri 360 GmbH
Ferdinand-Jühlke-Straße 7
99095 Erfurt, Deutschland
produktsicherheit@kolibri360.de

Druck:
CPI Druckdienstleistungen GmbH
im Auftrag der
Kolibri 360 GmbH
Ferdinand-Jühlke-Str. 7
99095 Erfurt